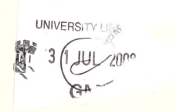

SOCIAL PROBLEMS AND SOCIAL ISSUES
An Aldine de Gruyter Series of Texts and Monographs
SERIES EDITOR
Joel Best, *University of Delaware*

Qualitative Methods and Health Policy Research

ELIZABETH MURPHY

ROBERT DINGWALL

ALDINE DE GRUYTER
New York

About the Authors

Elizabeth Murphy is Reader in Sociology and Social Policy at the University of Nottingham, United Kingdom.

Robert Dingwall is Professor and Director of the Institute for the Study of Genetics, Biorisks and Society at the University of Nottingham, United Kingdom.

ALDINE DE GRUYTER
A division of Walter de Gruyter, Inc.
200 Saw Mill River Road
Hawthorne, New York 10532

This publication is printed on acid free paper ∞

Library of Congress Cataloging-in-Publication Data

Murphy, Elizabeth.
    Qualitative methods and health policy research / Elizabeth Murphy and Robert Dingwall.
        p. cm.—(Social problems and social issues)
    Includes bibliographical references and index.
    ISBN 0-202-30710-7 1005260121
    1. Medical policy—Research—Methodology.   2. Qualitative research.   I. Dingwall, Robert. II. Title. III. Series.
    RA394.M87 2003
    362.1'07'2—dc21

                                                            2003001862

Manufactured in the United States of America

10 9 8 7 6 5 4 3 2 1

Contents

III   EVALUATING QUALITATIVE RESEARCH

Introduction

How can we possibly justify writing yet another book about qualitative research in health care? Are there not more than enough to satisfy the most discriminating researcher or methodology teacher? That may well be true but we think that there is a different kind of reader who needs a different kind of book. This is not another "how to do it" guide. We are writing for commissioners and consumers of health care research, those who have to plan, make policy, manage, and deliver services to, and for, sick people. Many of them have become increasingly aware that research based on qualitative methods could give them information that would not otherwise be available. This information would help them toward their goal of providing health care ever more efficiently, effectively, fairly, and compassionately. But these consumers are also confused by the apparent absence of the quality standards with which they are familiar from quantitative research. How can they decide whether the information offered to them is representative, valid, and reliable? What can they do with an approach that seems to be long on theory and short on facts?

The consumers' confusion is not helped by the disagreements between qualitative researchers themselves. Some qualitative researchers regard their work as a branch of the creative arts rather than as a form of policy science. This book does not oppose the liberal case for supporting scholarship in the humanities. However, it does question the claim of those who reject the model of policy science to be granted the privileges that go with it. In this respect, at least, it is also a book that we hope our peers will read as a manifesto for what in the United Kingdom we have come, under the influence of Martyn Hammersley (1992a), to call "subtle realism" and which U.S. scholars are beginning to defend as 'realist ethnography' (see Flaherty et al. 2002).

We shall explain what we mean by these terms as the book develops. Qualitative work does not have a *right* to any particular share of the research

1

dollar any more than it has a *right* to command the attention of consumers. It is the social scientist's responsibility to communicate clearly, not the reader's to struggle constantly with obscure or pretentious writing. If we can accomplish this, then we believe that the case for supporting qualitative work, and for discriminating between good and bad examples of it, will be compelling.

What is our status for writing this book? Between us we have over thirty years' experience of doing policy-oriented qualitative research in health care. We have walked the streets of major cities with public health nurses visiting mothers with young children. We have observed interdisciplinary teams discussing interventions in child abuse and neglect. We have sat in busy emergency rooms and watched family practitioners in their offices. We have talked to diabetics about why they do not take their medication or follow advice about changing their lifestyles. We have studied the delivery of care to people with back pain and the delivery of lifestyle advice to smokers. We have interviewed mothers and health professionals about child care practices. Our graduate students have looked at topics as diverse as organizational reforms in hospitals and primary care, the practice of surgery and anesthesia, and relations between minority women and obstetric care providers. In the course of our careers, we have used all the major technologies of qualitative research: observation, interviews, interaction analysis of audio or video recordings of clinical practice, and the analysis of images and documents. The direct inspiration for this book came from a commission from the UK National Health Service Health Technology Assessment Programme to write a report on the possible relevance of qualitative methods for their work. In the language of the moment, this book is a reimagining of that report (Murphy et al. 1998). Freed from the constraints of commissioned impartiality, we can set out our case for realist qualitative research as a branch of policy science and illustrate this through a review of major U.S. qualitative contributions to the social scientific study of health care.

We identify three kinds of research consumer in this book. Most of it is directed at those potential users who are agnostic, in the best sense of that word. They have not yet decided whether qualitative research has anything specific to offer them but are curious to know more about it and open to the possibility that they might find something useful in the course of this search. Those readers may prefer to go directly to Chapter 3. Before we get to the positive case, however, we have written two chapters for the other types of consumer. One of these is the sort of person who rejects any knowledge that does not come in quantitative form, believing this to be the only guarantee of the truth, objectivity, and disinterestedness of that information. The other is the sort who often claims to have some existing familiarity with qualitative research and is enthusiastic about it precisely because they believe that it introduces an element of humanity, subjectivity, and moral or political critique that is excluded by quantitative research. We think that both of these views are wrong and explain why.

We then take a more practical turn as we review each of the main qualitative research technologies. This book does not tell readers how to use these as researchers: rather, it explains what information each can generate, how that information can be evaluated, and how it can then feed into the improvement of health care planning, organization, or delivery.

Finally, we return to some more general statements. How can consumers recognize quality? How can they discriminate between good and bad examples of qualitative research? Where does qualitative research fit in the essential portfolio of evidence-based practice, management, or policy?

The earlier report, that forms the foundation of this book, was prepared in collaboration with David Greatbatch, Susan Parker, and Pamela Watson, and we would like to thank all of them for their contributions. The approach to social research outlined within it is the product of many years' reading and conversation with a large number of friends and colleagues. They include, but are not restricted to, David Altheide, J. Maxwell Atkinson, Paul Atkinson, David Armstrong, Howard Becker, Michael Bloor, Charles Bosk, Robert Emerson, Eliot Freidson, Harold Garfinkel, Jay Gubrium, Martyn Ham-mersley, John Heritage, Jim Holstein, the late Gordon Horobin, David Hughes, Veronica James, John M. Johnson, Peter Manning, Douglas Maynard, Gale Miller, Anne Murcott, Roger Murphy, Virginia Olesen, Susan Silbey, David Silverman, Gilbert Smith, the late Anselm Strauss, and the late Philip M. Strong. None of them, of course, are to blame for what follows. We should also like to acknowledge the specific comments of Martyn Hammersley and Alison Pilnick on sections of the present manuscript and the hospitality of the American Bar Foundation, where the copyedited text was ultimately prepared for the printer. Finally, we would like to commend Richard Koffler's patience with the delays imposed by career contingencies unforeseen when he first issued us with a contract and thank Mike Sola for his judicious copyediting.

I

The Contribution of Qualitative Research

1

Qualitative Research and Policy Science

What are your motives for reading this book? Are you a skeptic who believes that the only valid and reliable knowledge is that which comes in quantitative forms, and who wants to know why there is so much fuss about qualitative methods? Are you already a convert who believes that qualitative research is a way to bring romance back into a world that has been dulled by number crunching? Or are you an agnostic, who just wants to know whether there might be anything in this stuff that could be useful to you, your organization, and your patients? This chapter and the next are directed primarily at the first two readers. For the skeptic, they explain that qualitative research can be done in ways that are precise, rigorous, and scientific. For the romantic, they explain why many qualitative researchers have been reasserting the virtues of precision, rigor, and science against the recent fashion for subjectivity, empathy, and emotional politics. In the process, however, the agnostic will learn how we come to adopt the subtle realist foundations that underpin the remainder of this book.

Skeptical consumers frequently describe qualitative research with words like "soft," "impressionistic," "ideological," and "anecdotal." In context, these usually amount to a charge that the work is not scientific, as the skeptic understands that word. If qualitative research is not science, then it cannot contribute to a sound evidence base in health care policy and practice. Given this, it has nothing to offer to busy men and women concerned with the important practical issues of health service design, organization, and delivery. We disagree. We think that qualitative research can be done in a scientific fashion with rigor and precision. The means by which these are achieved may be unfamiliar to the skeptic but the objectives are identical.

As we set out a subtle realist program, however, we are conscious that this contradicts many features of some contemporary qualitative research that attract romantic consumers. They think this approach provides an element of color and humanity that has been eliminated by what they regard as the straitjacket of quantitative research. In their vocabulary, quantitative methods are "scientistic," "positivistic," "malestream," "artificial," "crushing of meaning," and so on. Their enthusiasm is fueled by sections of the qualitative research community. For example, the editors of the influential *Handbook of Qualitative Research* claim, in the latest edition, that the history of qualitative research in North America can be divided into seven phases or "moments." The current, sixth, moment is one in which "fictional ethnographies, ethnographic poetry, and multimedia texts are today taken for granted" (Denzin & Lincoln 2000:17). The barriers between scientific and other forms of writing, including journalism, fiction, and poetry, are being broken down (Ellis & Bochner 1996). Researchers are openly committed to "ideological research" that will contribute to the overthrow of patriarchy, neocolonialism, or global capitalism (Lather 1986). Qualitative research is to be understood as a "moral, allegorical, and therapeutic project" within which "the researcher's story is written as a prop, a pillar that … will help men and women endure and prevail in the dawning years of the 21st century" (Denzin & Lincoln 2000:xvi). These approaches are claimed to be as acceptable as more traditional ones: "There can be no question that the legitimacy of postmodern paradigms is well established and at least equal to the legitimacy of received and conventional paradigms" (Lincoln & Guba 2000:164).

In the context of this romantic turn, the skeptics' reaction to qualitative research is understandable, and we share a great deal of it. However, it makes our task more difficult, in that we must explain both why we think that qualitative research can offer useful knowledge for policy and practice and why we do not think that the search for alternative standards from the humanities is helpful. In the words of one early critic of this turn, we think that it is more important to be "right" than to be "right-on" (Strong 1988). This chapter looks at three issues where the pressure from romantics gives skeptics most cause for concern:

- Is qualitative research science?
- Can qualitative research reports be distinguished from journalism or fiction?
- Is qualitative research driven by a political agenda rather than by a quest for useful knowledge?

We shall show that realist qualitative researchers need not abandon a commitment to science or the search for authoritative knowledge. We do not believe that the dissolution of the boundaries between scientific and other kinds of writing is helpful. Finally, we believe that seeing research as primarily a political project confuses the roles of knowledge producer and activist in ways that are unhelpful and that undermine research's potential contribution to practical social change.

QUALITATIVE RESEARCH AS SCIENCE

Qualitative researchers have traditionally been cautious about claiming that their work was scientific. The "right-on" schools have exaggerated this caution into an outright rejection of science as a model for their work. Science is, for them, outmoded, "an archaic form of consciousness surviving for a while yet in a degraded form" (Tyler 1986:200). Scientists' assertions that they are in pursuit of truth simply camouflage their own lust for power. There is no essential difference between truth and propaganda. "Truth games" are represented as a form of terrorism (Rosenau 1992). The result is sometimes described as a *crisis of legitimation*, that there is no form of knowledge that is not arbitrary, subjective, and biased by interests (Lincoln & Guba 2000).

The boundary between science and propaganda has often been breached (Fay 1996) and some distrust of scientific claims may certainly be healthy (Sanders 1995). However, just because we can find examples of propaganda masquerading as science and of science being exploited as propaganda, it does not follow that propaganda and science are synonymous. Similarly, we can question the claim that science creates disinterested and objective knowledge of an observer-independent world without concluding that science is impossible.

The skeptics' reservations about qualitative research are usually based on the deep-rooted assumption among natural scientists, and some social scientists, that there is a world "out there," prior to, and independent of, their observations. This world can be known objectively in the sense that all observers will, if identically placed, see it in exactly the same way. If a suitable language were available, they would also all produce identical descriptions. From these observations they can work out the laws governing the world's operations. Truth is simply a matter of correct description. Particular observations and statements of laws might contain errors but these will be corrected by further data or better observational techniques. Neither observations nor laws have any moral or ethical implication: they simply describe what is. The consumer of science is, ideally, presented with a structured set of facts and the laws that describe the relationship between these facts. If A is necessary for B and C to happen, then preventing A from happening will eliminate B and C.

If we take medicine as an example, this model would lead to the view that human diseases have always and everywhere been the same, at least once established in the species. If they have been described and classified in different ways by different cultures or at different historical periods, this is because there has been insufficient systematic data to establish their true nature. As this is collected, universally valid descriptions will be produced. In principle, then, any doctor seeing a patient with a particular disease will, if not today then at some foreseeable point in the future, see the same disease and describe it in the same terms. From being a "catchall" term for uncontrolled cellular growths, for instance, many specialists now talk of "cancer" as the aggregate of possibly several hundred different diseases, whose individual characters are gradually being captured and defined. We may look back in a hundred years' time, as we now look back to the nineteenth-century disease of chlorosis, to a disease category that was once widely used and is now extinct (Figlio 1978). However, this is a sign of progress, of a closer approximation to the truth of disease replacing our current errors. Whatever names we give to these new disease categories, they have always been there: it is simply that we can now see them properly.

Although this approach has resulted in many valuable contributions to the welfare of humankind, it has never gone unquestioned. Ever since philosophers began debating the nature of science more than two thousand years ago, there has been a competing view that the world "out there" is shaped and organized, if not actually created, by the perceptions of the observer. In consequence, claims to know that world objectively must be treated with caution. Knowledge always rests on some point of view—on some mixture of the observer's prior knowledge, experience, values, and motives with their biological and technological capacities. All facts are *artifacts*, products of the processes by which we decide what might be important to notice and record and of the concepts that frame those processes. In Fay's words, "Descriptions always take place *within* a framework which provides the conceptual resources in and through which reality (or events and objects in it) is described" (1996:74). This framework is not, however, purely subjective. At the most basic level, one of the ways in which we constantly affirm our sanity is by seeing the world in the way expected of ordinary members of the social groups to which we belong (Goffman 1983). If we see a fuzzy road sign, we *know* that our vision is at fault rather than the sign (Pollner 1975). As scholars, we usually show our competence by demonstrating that we see the world in the way that people with our particular training and status would be expected to.

Natural scientists, then, have to learn a specific way of seeing the world in order to be accepted as competent in their field. This is enforced by the social processes of recruitment, organization, and control within the scientific community. If disease categories, such as "cancer," vary over time, this does not show a progressive approximation to the essential truth of nature but the consequences of changes within the scientific community. Different generations use different investigative technologies and different classificatory criteria, associated with different therapies and different goals. The underlying biological structures and processes are seen through different frames, giving them a different appearance. The change from one frame to another over time is rarely a matter of truth correcting error but rather of changing ideas about what would count as truth and error. There might, indeed, be a real world out there somewhere: we can, however, only know it through a process that is subject to both social and psychological influences. The results can amalgamate statements of fact and statements of value. When we say that "X is a disease," for example, we are not just describing X but also communicating a value judgment about X, that it is undesirable (Dingwall 2001). Conversely, a negative evaluation of X might lead to its, apparently factual, classification as a disease. Think, for example, of the long-running debate within the American Psychiatric Association about whether or not homosexuality should be defined as a disease that the profession should seek to "cure" (Bayer 1987).

Some qualitative researchers have gone on from this to conclude that they should give up any claim to be doing science and adopt some form of relativism (Ellis & Flaherty 1992; Lather 1993). Relativists assert that we decide what counts as "real" *only* through the linguistic and cultural resources of the groups to which we belong, which frame our interaction with the world (Fay 1996). Consequently, it is possible for many different realities to exist or even for there to be as many realities as there are persons (Smith 1984:386). Individual realities may contradict one another and yet still be equally true for those operating within them. We cannot test such realities against "objective facts" since "facts" are themselves produced by reference to conceptual frameworks. In a discussion of witchcraft and psychotherapy, Fay (1996) illustrates the difficulties that result. Relativists cannot distinguish between psychotherapy and witchcraft as means of dealing with strange behavior. The prior decision, whether to believe in witchcraft or in psychotherapy, shapes the very perception of what behavior will be counted as strange and how it can properly be explained. Claims about the world are only true, if the idea of truth has any meaning at all, within the frameworks adopted by those who make the claims. In that sense, all claims to truth are arbitrary.

The relativist position denies that there is any independent basis on which we can choose between different conceptual frameworks or the realities they produce. There is no possibility of a "God's eye point of view" (Smith 1985). Standards of judgment are internal to particular conceptual schemes, so they cannot be applied across them. There is no way to evaluate the adequacy of one explanation or description against another. Relativists turn, instead, to moral, ethical, or political criteria. Truth claims rest on moral superiority or political expediency, on being "right-on" rather than being "right." Research illustrates or justifies a prior position, which is itself placed beyond question. For romantic consumers of qualitative research, this is part of its attraction, that it can sustain what they already believe.

For skeptical consumers, however, such relativism further undermines the usefulness of qualitative research for practice (Greene 1996; Sanders 1995). If researchers' only possible output is one more story, one more reality among an indefinite number of possible realities, what good are they? Why should they expect financial support in competition with novelists, poets, or artists (Strong 1983)? The public funding of research and scholarship rests on an implicit contract to produce knowledge that is in some sense relevant to the goals and values of a society (Hammersley 1995). Relativism undermines the foundations of that contract.

The relativists' conclusion can be criticized in a number of ways. First, it is self-refuting. If the claim that all truths are relative is true, then this claim itself must be relative. The claim can only be true in terms of a particular set of assumptions that others may judge to be false. Second, it certainly underestimates the extent to which reality has a way of resisting our constructions. The world we observe has the crucial ability to "talk back" (Dawson & Prus 1995). While it may be true that any observation is irreducibly an interpretation of the world, it is not true that the world will bear any interpretation we care to put upon it. Garfinkel (2002:173–5) has recently characterized this as "natural accountability," the challenge to produce descriptions that are above all disciplined by the local particulars of the "shop floor," the material and cognitive environment in which real things happen. "The obdurate character of the empirical world" (Blumer 1969:22) can challenge our conceptual frameworks. Would you want to fly straight and level at five thousand feet from Denver to San Francisco with a pilot who thought the Rockies were a social construct? Even a postmodernist cannot play football with a broken leg. Third, it creates an implausible model of social organization. It leads to the claim that different people inhabit different and incommensurable worlds with no possibility of meaningful communication between them. If this were correct, human social interaction would be literally impossible, since there would be no common reference points.

Relativism is not the only possible response to the loose coupling between the world and our understanding of it. An alternative, which we argue is more appropriate for policy science, is what Hammersley (1992a) has called "subtle realism." This acknowledges that researchers are constrained by the prior frames that they bring to their observations (Hammersley & Atkinson 1995). The observer's knowledge is, however, always "a *joint* product of the referent and the cultural-biological lenses through which it [the phenomenon under study] is seen" (Campbell 1994:157, emphasis added). The subtle realist accepts that a world exists independently of its observers and constrains the observations that can be made. At the same time those observations are also constrained by the "cultural-biological lens" through which they are made.

Subtle realists accept that everything can be represented from a range of different perspectives, through different "cultural-biological lenses." Several representations may coexist and be potentially true. Unlike the relativist, however, the subtle realist does not assume that all these representations are equally valid. Judgments can be made about their truth or falsity. We may never know with absolute certainty that a particular knowledge claim is true (Hammersley 1993). Nevertheless, claims can be rigorously tested and evaluated. We can make a judgment about whether they are adequately supported by evidence and argument. Dewey referred to this as "warranted assertability" (1938:7), while Phillips talks about "truth as a regulative ideal" (1987:23).

Science, in this view, is a *procedural* commitment. In practice, it consists of openness to refutation, a conscientious and systematic search for contradictory evidence, and a readiness to subject one's preconceptions to critical examination. The devotion to truth as a regulative ideal is an essential difference between science and propaganda. Through its natural accountability, science is always capable of being changed by inconvenient data. Propaganda merely seeks to ignore, incorporate or explain away contradictory evidence. As such, objectivity is above all an attitude or "a state of mind," which can characterize any kind of research. Qualitative research regulated by an ideal of truth should be capable of satisfying skeptical consumers that it meets their basic tests of science, even if the specific means adopted are unfamiliar. The next chapter will describe some of the general characteristics of the procedural commitments that we advocate for qualitative research.

QUALITATIVE RESEARCH AND FORMS OF WRITING

Skeptical consumers frequently charge qualitative research reports with being indistinguishable from forms of writing like journalism and fiction. Ironically, many contemporary qualitative researchers would take this as praise rather than as criticism. As we have seen, they reject conventional forms of scientific writing as part of their program to break down the boundaries between science and the humanities (Ellis & Bochner 1996; Richardson 1988, 1992). These researchers have turned to alternative forms of writing in an attempt to escape the rhetoric, epistemology, and politics of conventional research reporting. Textual innovations include poetry

(Austin 1996; Richardson 1992; Tillmann-Healy 1996), collage (Clifford 1981), personal narratives (Ronai 1992, 1996; Tillman-Healy 1996; Ellis 1996; Kolker 1996), dramatic presentations and constructed dialogues (Bluebond-Langer 1980; Ellis & Bochner 1992; Mienczakowski & Morgan 1993; Paget 1990), and polyvocal texts (Fox 1996). These experiments respond to what is described as the *crisis of representation*, because it arises from self-conscious questioning of what counts as an adequate representation of reality (Richardson 1988).

The advocates of these alternative writing forms are dissatisfied with conventional research reports on three grounds. The first is aesthetic: conventional reports are accused of being "dreary" (Richardson 1992), "formulaic" (Richardson 1988), or "boring, esoteric and parochial" (Ellis & Bochner 1996). In particular, they focus on the cognitive at the expense of the emotional (Ellis & Bochner 1996). The second is closely linked to the relativist position discussed above. Traditional forms of research report assume that there is an independent and external reality to write about. If that assumption is rejected, then it is not surprising to find the rejection of the rhetorically impersonal and objective forms of writing that reflect it. The third objection is essentially political. Given their insistence that what we take to be reality is constituted through our own interpretive activity, many postmodernists question the right of researchers to impose their interpretations of reality on the people they study. The authors of "scientific" research reports usurp the authority of those people to speak for themselves. Alternative forms of writing are claimed to overcome some or all of these alleged shortcomings. First, such writing will be more accessible and interesting. Second, textual radicalism is a way of breaking down the distinction between observer and observed (Tyler 1986), disrupting and displacing the rhetorical devices that establish the researcher's authority at the expense of those under study (Lather 1991). Finally, certain kinds of experimental writing, particularly the presentation of unedited interview transcripts, without analysis or theorizing, are a means of "giving voice" to those being studied in a way that is otherwise denied to them.

The responsibility for effective communication is not entirely one-sided. Different kinds of writing call for different types of engagement from readers. Whether or not a text is boring or dreary depends, to a certain extent, upon the expectations that are brought by readers. If readers approach scientific research reports with the same expectations as they bring to reading novels or glossy magazines then they are indeed likely to be disappointed. Nevertheless, it is undeniable that some conventional social scientific writing is boring and dreary. However, it is equally the case that some is well-written and compelling. Moreover, the experimental writing, with which critics seek to replace it, is not universally faultless. As Sanders comments, "Postmodernists frequently stumble and produce materials

that read like high-school creative writing exercises or passages from me-
diocre cyberpunk novels" (1995:95). He argues that much of what is produced in such genres tends to be intensely narcissistic. At worst, it
"represents lengthy therapeutic rambling in which the writer insists upon
telling us about his or her dreams, personal insecurities, 'meditations,' and
sources of 'panic'" (ibid.:96). While such accounts may have a certain voy-
euristic fascination, they can become just as dreary as poor reporting in a
more conventional style. If we want readers to be interested in what we
write, then we must write as interestingly and engagingly as possible.
Experimental forms do not guarantee success in this respect any more than
do conventional approaches.

The second objection begins from the observation that conventional
authors purport to report on the reality of what they have witnessed in a
setting or discovered through talking to those who are the object of study.
For relativists, however, reality does not exist before its observation. Researchers, therefore, actually produce the reality they appear to be describing through their writing. This productive activity is hidden from the reader
by the range of rhetorical devices commonly used in so-called realist texts.
As a result, readers are deceived into treating these texts as objective reports
rather than as subjective creations.

The authors of such reports, for example, are generally completely absent from the texts they produce. Such "writing out of the author from the
text" can be observed in many early anthropological and sociological works
(e.g., Malinowski 1922; Evans-Pritchard 1940; Becker, Geer, Hughes, &
Strauss 1961). It is achieved through linguistic devices such as the use of
the passive voice and a neutral, authoritative tone. These have the effect
of creating what Richardson terms "an illusion of objectivity" (1988:203).
Richardson describes the consequences of this authorial self-effacement:

> The implied narrator is godlike, an all-knowing voice from afar and above,
> stripped of all human subjectivity and fallibility. But, in fact, science does have
> a human narrator, the "camouflaged first person," hiding in the bramble of
> the passive voice. (ibid.:203)

The impression created is one of "immaculate perception" (Van Maanen
1988), which disguises the author's preconceptions. This is not just one of
a number of possible versions: it is *the* version.

The status of conventional reports may also be bolstered by appeals to
the experiential authority of the researcher. In effect, the researcher says to
the reader, "I was there, so I should know." Seale (1999) shows how the
confessional narratives or "tales from the field," which are included in many
qualitative research monographs, serve the purpose of asserting the
author's privileged claim to *know* the setting under study. Superficially,

these confessional tales often report on the researcher's initial mistakes and failures. They typically present these as part of a learning experience that allows the author to improve their technique and overcome barriers to gaining an insider's understanding of the setting. As such, they reinforce the privileged authority of the researcher's account. Similarly, the inclusion of a great deal of description of the mundane details of the research setting in many qualitative reports emphasizes the researcher's so-called privilege of presence (Dawson & Prus 1995) and underwrites his or her claim to authoritative knowledge.

Strategies like these are said to obscure the socially constructed nature of research reports. This links them to the third objection to conventional reporting forms. Here, the argument is a political one—that the rhetorical strategies employed in scientific reports obscure not just the theoretical but also the ideological nature of researchers' activities. Under the cloak of objectivity, researchers impose their own point of view, silencing the voices of those who are the objects of their study (Clifford 1986; Denzin & Lincoln 1994). Fine describes this as "a colonizing discourse of the Other" (1994:70). Authority to represent the other, and hence to define what will count as reality about the other, is recognized as one of the ways in which power relationships are played out (Kleinman 1993). The colonialist, sexist, and elitist assumptions embedded in much qualitative research reporting are cited as evidence of the way in which such writing is inherently conservative.

It is important to recognize that all research reports are inescapably "artful products" (Atkinson 1990:2), employing a range of rhetorical and textual strategies. They must be approached with critical sensitivity to the devices that are being used both to advance an argument and to persuade the reader of its merits. Scientific reports are not immaculately conceived reproductions of reality (Charmaz 1995). They are, at best, "partial truths" (Clifford 1986). Any account, scientific or otherwise, is necessarily selective in that it highlights certain aspects of reality, as seen from certain perspectives, and ignores or downplays others (Sanders 1995). The selectivity and potential bias of researcher interpretations do raise important political issues.

However, the problems may not be inevitable or the proposed solutions helpful. As subtle realists, we do not start from the denial of an external world that drives the position outlined above. Since we accept that the settings and people we study are real, it is entirely consistent to try to represent them as accurately as possible when we write about them. Our representations will always be partial, and will sometimes be mistaken, but our objective in writing can be to present as full and faithful a picture as we possibly can. This is what is meant by treating truth as a regulative ideal. Where the goal of postmodernist writing may be evocation, ours continues to be the accurate representation of the phenomena we study.

Treating truth as a regulative ideal has profound implications for the ways in which we write about our research findings. We must present our findings and arguments, and the evidence we call upon to support them, as clearly and precisely as possible. Clarity opens up the possibilities of challenge and refutation that are central to science. As Hammersley (1995:95) argues, the preeminent requirement of any scientific report is that it should lay itself open to rational assessment of the validity of its knowledge claims. We should certainly examine the appropriateness of the interpretations that researchers make of the data they collect, asking to what extent alternative interpretations have been sought and evaluated (Dawson & Prus 1995). Unlike those who argue that the function of qualitative research is to give voice to the oppressed, we believe that our commitment should be to ensuring that, as far as possible, voices at all levels of the organizations and settings we study are incorporated into our analyses. We shall discuss precisely how these objectives might be accomplished in Chapters 7 and 9. Anything that obscures the line of argument, or confuses the evidence upon which that argument is based, should be resisted. This applies equally to "realist tales," which hide from view the author's role in generating and interpreting data, and to radical textual strategies, whose authors deliberately reject both faithful representation and rational argument. Art and literature both play an important role in society. They may evoke aspects of human experience that are resistant to scientific investigation. Such evocations may have enormous potential for stimulating desirable change but they should not be confused with science.

THE POLITICAL AGENDA OF QUALITATIVE RESEARCH

A final common criticism that is frequently leveled at qualitative research by skeptics relates to its supposedly political nature. Once again, there is some basis for this. Just as many qualitative researchers have tried to move closer to the humanities, so many (often the same ones) have tried to erode the boundaries between research and politics. Their avowed goal is to promote emancipation from sources of domination and repression rather than to produce knowledge (Anderson 1989; Gitlin, Siegel, & Boru 1989; Harding 1987). The intended beneficiaries of such emancipation include women, ethnic or racial minorities, gay men and women, and the working class. For example, Richardson (1988) defines her research task as one that is primarily political. Her responsibility is to "help construct a consciousness of kind in the minds of the protagonists, a concrete recognition of sociological bondedness with others, because such consciousness can break down isolation between people, empower them, and lead to collective action on their behalf" (ibid.:201). The inability of traditional forms of qualitative research to achieve this is seen as a *crisis of praxis* (Lincoln & Guba 2000).

It is, of course, true that all research, whether qualitative or quantitative, is in some sense political, even when it does not acknowledge this. Hammersley (1995) discusses the range of ways in which research can be said to be colored by politics. Social research always involves power relationships with those who are being researched, although it would be simplistic to assume that, in such relationships, power is exercised exclusively by researchers at the expense of those being studied (Murphy & Dingwall 2001). Research participants have considerable scope for exerting power over researchers (Hammersley 1992c; Lincoln 1990). It is also true that research is necessarily value-laden. All research involves selecting and giving priority to some goal or goals at the expense of others: the choice of goal implies some kind of value judgment. As Hammersley (1995) argues, even if we understand the goal of research to be that of producing knowledge, then this presupposes that knowledge is preferable to ignorance. Similarly the choice of one topic rather than another, whether by investigators or sponsors, is value-laden, as are the decisions of the gatekeepers who grant access to particular research settings. Researchers' presuppositions are inevitably to some extent shaped by the culture and values of the various groups to which they belong. Research can—and does—have material consequences both for those studied and for the groups of which they are a part (Murphy & Dingwall 2001). In all these senses, all research is a value-laden and, arguably, a political activity.

However, there is a considerable difference between accepting that all research is value-laden and arguing that the aim of research should be to promote political change, or, for that matter, political stability. Unlike those qualitative researchers who commit themselves to furthering political goals through their research, we believe that the primary goal of research should be the pursuit of knowledge and the limitation of error. Researchers have no particular license that entitles them to draw prescriptive conclusions from their findings. If we confuse the role of political activist with that of researcher, we run the risk of undermining the distinction between science and polemic that is the basis of our claim to have something to say to decision-makers. We shall return to this topic in Chapter 8.

CONCLUSION

Policy science calls for research that is committed to the pursuit of knowledge and the elimination of error. It proceeds through the rigorous development, refinement, and testing of knowledge claims. It emphasizes clarity and precision in the presentation of findings. In this way it opens itself to challenge and refutation. It can, and should, make a contribution that is distinct from, and yet complementary to, that of the arts and the humanities. That contribution will be enhanced where qualitative researchers are mindful of their role as generators of knowledge rather than as champions of political goals. This is the vision of qualitative research that we develop in this book.

2

Three Myths about Qualitative Research

In the previous chapter we showed that qualitative research is a highly contested field, riddled with claims and counterclaims about its fundamental assumptions. It is not, however, necessary to accept the conclusions that romantic authors and consumers have drawn from postmodern and ideological critiques of traditional practice. Later in the book, we shall develop our alternative arguments, that it is still perfectly possible to carry out scientific inquiry, to describe this in a reasonably disinterested fashion, and to apply the results to the benefit of humankind. Before doing so, however, we need to clear some further ground. In particular, we shall explore in more detail some of the issues that we touched on previously in discussing what it would mean to do qualitative research in a scientific way. What makes qualitative research legitimate?

We do this by confronting three myths that have grown up around qualitative research to justify the claim by both skeptics and romantics that it is in some profound way radically different from quantitative research. These myths assert that qualitative research depends upon different forms of logical reasoning, that it is more natural, and that it gives direct access to the meaning of actions for the people who take part in them. For the skeptics, this combination justifies the exclusion of qualitative research from the community of science, to which quantitative work is admitted. If these commentators recognize any role at all for qualitative research, it is a relatively minor one (see, for example, Imle & Atwood 1988). At best, they tend to think that qualitative research may be helpful in preparatory work before "real science" is undertaken. Like the skeptics, the romantics hold that qualitative research is fundamentally different from quantitative research but they then assert that it is actually these differences that make it a superior way of understanding the social world.

20

MYTH NUMBER ONE: QUALITATIVE RESEARCH IS INDUCTIVE

The first myth is that the logic underpinning qualitative research is fundamentally different from that which is found in quantitative research. This supposed distinction is expressed in various ways. Sometimes qualitative research is said to be "theory-generating" by comparison with "theory-testing" quantitative research. Readers are frequently told that qualitative research is concerned with discovery, where quantitative research is committed to verification. However, these are essentially only different ways of saying that qualitative research relies on induction rather than deduction (Shaffir, Stebbins, & Turowetz 1980; Imle & Atwood 1988; Merriam 1988; Habermann-Little 1991; Munhall 1993; Morse 1994).

A deductive research strategy starts with theory, from which hypotheses are derived. These hypotheses are subsequently defined in terms of the processes of measurement that are used to test them through empirical investigations. A health care manager may have a theory that consumer satisfaction is related to the length of time that patients have to wait on her service. This can be stated as the hypothesis that there is a negative association between the duration of waiting and consumer satisfaction, that is, reducing waiting times increases satisfaction with a service. We may have some general ideas about what consumer satisfaction might be, but we can only measure changes if we turn it into a rating scale. Such a scale should be a good reflection of our underlying idea (validity) and capable of being scored in a reasonably consistent fashion by different people who use it (reliability). "Consumer satisfaction," for this purpose, is what is measured by our rating scale. This process of conversion is called "operationalization."[1]

Of course, myths are rarely entirely without foundation. Qualitative researchers have been at the forefront of moves to rehabilitate induction as a proper activity for scientists. It is important to recognize that induction is not the same as intuition or empathy, with which it is frequently confused in some romantic approaches. Inductive research starts with empirical data and proceeds systematically to infer general principles or theoretical statements. The nineteenth-century English philosopher John Stuart Mill produced the most influential formal specification of induction's underlying logic (Mill 1973). This involves four methods: the method of *agreement*, where apparently different cases with similar outcomes are examined to see what material feature they have in common; the method of *difference*, where apparently similar cases with different outcomes are examined to see in what material respect they actually differ; the method of *residues*, where the contribution of known factors is subtracted from the outcome so that what is left must represent the outstanding material contribution; and the method of *concomitant variation*, where the simultaneous variation of two outcomes suggests that a link can be found between them, that one causes the other, or that they are both caused by the same underlying factor. Of course, as with any methodology, this has technical difficulties in knowing that all features have been examined, in determining what is and is not a material feature, in separating causation and correlation. The point, however, is that induction is not an unsystematic or occult process. There is a formal logic to be followed.

The key text in the revival of induction by qualitative researchers is often taken to be Glaser and Strauss's (1967) *The Discovery of Grounded Theory*. The authors were critical of the narrow preoccupation with theory testing that characterized social research in the 1960s. Critical rationalists, influenced particularly by Popper (1959), had argued that only deductive research could be characterized as scientific. At best, inductive strategies were "pseudoscientific." For Popper, the essence of science was hypothesis testing. He disassociated science from any concern about the source of hypotheses:

> The initial stage, the act of conceiving or inventing a theory, seems to me neither to call for logical analysis nor to be susceptible to it. The question of how it happens that a new idea occurs to a man—whether it is a musical theme, a dramatic conflict, or a scientific theory—may be of great interest to empirical psychology; but it is irrelevant to the logical analysis of scientific knowledge. (ibid.:31–32)

This obsession with rigorous deductive theorizing and testing led researchers to neglect the equally important task of theory generation. Glaser and Strauss urged social scientists to turn their attention to generating theory that was grounded in empirical reality.

Qualitative research was a central means by which such data-grounded theory could be developed. Given the limited resources available to support scientific work, it is hardly surprising that practicing researchers try to concentrate their efforts on those theories that are most likely to be viable. Perhaps if the context for health researchers offered infinite resources and no time constraints, then the source of our hypotheses would indeed be immaterial. With enough hard work, intuition, and good luck, we could expect eventually to come up with hypotheses that would move our knowledge forward. The strict Popperian model has something in common with the idea that a sufficient number of monkeys typing randomly at a sufficient number of keyboards for long enough would ultimately reproduce the works of Shakespeare. However, in our environment, resources are limited and time is pressing. The rigorous testing of hypotheses, using either qualitative or quantitative methods, is expensive and time-consuming. It is necessary to be selective in identifying those hypotheses that are most likely to "fit" and "work" (Glaser & Strauss 1967).

In the forty years since this program was elaborated, it has inevitably acquired some accretions and misunderstandings of its own. An important one is an overemphasis on *discovery*, with an insistence on a fresh induction for each piece of research. This was understandable in the context of the 1960s when there was only a small body of empirical work using qualitative methods and each new study was likely to break fresh ground. However, while this remains a useful injunction, it understates the growing potential for cumulative work that builds systematically on previous studies. This is partly due to the neglect of the deductive elements in Glaser and Strauss's work. Indeed, in a later publication, Strauss acknowledged that both deductive and inductive thinking are central to grounded theory (Strauss & Corbin 1990). Qualitative research may begin from induction but proceeds to the development of theories that can be tested deductively, at least in the sense that they enable predictions to be made and natural experiments to be identified in which these pre-dictions can be examined. This movement backward and forward between theory and data is characteristic of much qualitative research (Emerson 1983).

The balance between induction and deduction varies across different qualitative research studies. Many do give priority to theory generation, while others emphasize theory testing. Indeed, as Lofland argued, much qualitative research is "simultaneously deductive and inductive" (1976:66). In qualitative work data analysis is rarely treated as a discrete stage of research. It occurs in parallel with data collection so that the researcher is continuously able to test, refine, and elaborate propositions developed in earlier stages of the research. Theoretical statements are modified in the light of new observations and observations are sought to extend or modify existing or emerging theory. Three examples illustrate this interplay between deduction and induction in different qualitative research studies.

Monica Casper's study of the emergence of fetal surgery, *The Making of the Unborn Patient*, emphasized theory generation: "From the outset, this project was envisioned as an ethnography designed to build theory from the ground up" (1998:18). She describes how the focus of her research emerged from her empirical work: "As I began observing fetal surgery, interviewing people, and attending staff meetings medical work itself emerged as the heart of the dynamics in which I was interested" (ibid.). It seems, then, that Casper did not approach her research topic with a pre-formulated set of hypotheses to be tested. Her approach is represented as one of approaching her research setting with a blank mind and allowing her research to be driven by whatever emerged from her observations, rather than by any preconceived ideas or theoretical frameworks. On closer examination, however, it becomes apparent that her analyses are actually the product of a careful interweaving of existing theory and her own observations. In particular, she began to understand the social organization of the Fetal Treatment Unit in relation to the work of Strauss and his coinvestigators (1964) on the negotiated order of psychiatric hospitals. This theoretical framework may not have been imposed upon her data through the formal generation of testable hypotheses. Nevertheless, the study involved the examination of the fit between Strauss's theory and the interactions and work practices she observed in the unit. As a result, much of the reported observation and analysis can be seen to involve testing hypotheses derived from Strauss even though the testing is generally more informal than formal. Casper's account is, then, as much one of theory elaboration through testing as of theory generation.

The second example differs insofar as the authors explicitly identify their study as an attempt at hypothesis testing. David Silverman and his coresearchers analyzed the organization and reception of advice-giving in human immunodeficiency virus (HIV) counseling sessions (Silverman et al. 1992). Their study was informed by earlier research on advice-giving in interactions between health professionals and mothers of young children (Heritage & Sefi 1992). In that study, Heritage and Sefi had found that most advice sequences were initiated by the health professional rather than by the mother. They identified four distinct forms of advice giving that occurred in these interactions. One of these four forms—stepwise entry—appeared to be associated with less resistance and more engagement by mothers. Stepwise entry involved the professional first eliciting a statement from the intended advice-recipient, the mother, identifying the problem that she was experiencing, or could experience, to which the advice would be directed. This statement might be further elaborated before the advice was actually delivered. In effect, skillful professionals managed to get the mothers to ask for the advice the professionals had intended to give them all along. Silverman and his coworkers derived a number of hypotheses from Heritage and Sefi's work and sought to test them in the context of HIV counseling sessions. Their data appeared to confirm Heritage and Sefi's findings. They found clear correlations between the form of advice-giving and the responses from clients. Where the counselor gave advice without eliciting a problem statement from the client, the client only showed a positive response to the advice in three cases out of the thirty-two analyzed. By contrast, in only four of the eighteen cases where advice was given following a client request, whether volunteered or elicited, did the response not indicate some engagement.

Silverman's study was designed to be hypothesis testing. The hypotheses were grounded in data insofar as they had been generated from earlier empirical work in different settings. Studies such as this reflect the growing legitimacy of hypothesis testing in qualitative research. This does not conflict with the agenda set by Glaser and Strauss (1967) in the 1960s. Their target was speculative or armchair theorizing. Thanks, in no small measure, to them, there is now a considerable body of theory that is grounded in empirical reality and open to testing, refinement, and elaboration. This has strengthened the opportunities for cumulative work as the theories generated in one setting or context are tested in another.

In some ways, this resembles the classic logic of experimental research as theory proposed on the basis of work in one context is tested against data derived from another context that is believed to differ in certain ways. The new findings either confirm or revise those of the first study. In their work on emergency rooms, for example, Dingwall and Murray (1983) brought together findings from three previous studies in the United Kingdom that demonstrated the negative treatment of certainly socially stigmatized groups. Writers like Sudnow (1967) and Roth and Douglas (1983) report similar findings from the United States. Dingwall and Murray adopted an explicitly Popperian approach. They formulated a model set of rules that had been identified in an influential previous study (Jeffery 1979) as the sources of authority for sanctioning stigmatized patients. However, when applied to the child patients in their study, the predicted sanctions were not observed, and so the model was rejected. From the results, they induced a more elaborate account of the reasoning of the medical and nursing staff in classifying patients and showed how this was related to the organizational contingencies of their work rather than to simple kinds of class, moral, or other prejudices. The understanding of the impact of organizational contingencies has been extended in recent work by Dodier and Camus (1998) in France. They show how the staffing of the service by residents covering from other specialties, rather than spending time in emergency work as part of a planned rotation or career choice, modifies the classificatory practices. These data from three countries can be brought together and shown to display certain common underlying features, which can, in principle, be used to make predictions about emergency work in other hospitals in other countries. The resource for the service manager is not the specific descriptions of practice in the United Kingdom, the United States, or France: rather, it is a cumulative understanding of the issues that arise in emergency work and of the roots of these issues in the organization of medical and nursing work and careers.

We have argued that the representation of qualitative research as inductive rather than deductive is misleading. This may be equally true of the claim that the logic of quantitative research is wholly deductive. The preoccupation with deduction is often linked to an aspiration to emulate the natural sciences. As we have seen, Popper's argument, that only deduction could be the basis for science, has been highly influential. However, as Lincoln and Guba (1985) observed, Popper's restrictive definition of science would exclude much of Einstein's work. Many working scientists prefer the model put forward by Wallace (1978). He argued that science involves both induction (via empirical generalizations) and deduction, leading to the testing of hypotheses. This process is circular, rather than linear, in that observations are synthesized into empirical generalizations, which can then be synthesized into theory. The resultant theory can be tested through the deduction of hypotheses, which are, in turn, subjected to further empirical observation. This is, in effect, the same process that Glaser and Strauss described.

In practice, quantitative research involves both deduction and induction. The separation of data collection and data analysis in quantitative research makes it less likely that a single study will involve both hypothesis generation and hypothesis testing. However, it is quite common for a program of research to involve both elements. Early descriptive work may inform the generation of hypotheses to be tested in later stages of the research. Moreover, some kinds of quantitative analysis are grounded in an inductive logic. In particular, both cluster and factor analysis, which seek to identify the dimensions of a phenomenon on the basis of the clustering of data, are clearly inductive techniques. Indeed, Schwandt (1997) has argued that the whole basis of probability theory is inductive, insofar as it involves moving from data on individual cases to claims about all cases.

The myth that there is a fundamental difference in the logic underlying qualitative and quantitative research has two unfortunate consequences. On the one hand, it makes a creative alliance between those working in different methodological traditions more difficult. On the other, it narrows the potential of qualitative research. By restricting its role to theory generation, qualitative research's potential contribution to cumulative knowledge building is thwarted.

MYTH NUMBER TWO: QUALITATIVE RESEARCH IS NATURAL

The second myth is that qualitative research is "natural." By implication, quantitative research is characterized as "artificial." Indeed the terms "naturalism" and "naturalistic" have often been used as synonyms for qualitative research (e.g., Lofland 1967; Denzin 1971; Schatzman & Strauss 1973; Lincoln & Guba 1985). Originally, the analogy was probably being made with "natural history," the study of living things in their own environments. In the context of the romantic program, however, "natural" and "artificial" are rarely used as neutral terms. As in many other areas of our contemporary culture, from organic foodstuffs to self-expression, the natural is equated with the good and the virtuous. The artificial is distorting, damaging, and even oppressive.

Again there is, of course, some truth to this myth. Qualitative researchers do emphasize the value of studying naturally occurring settings, of a "natural history" of human social organization. For example, when Guillemin and Holmstrom (1986) investigated intensive care facilities for newborn infants, they chose to do so by close observation of the units' day-to-day organization and functioning. They selected one "Level III" neonatal intensive care unit (i.e., a unit that provided maximum-level care) and, in their terms, "entered the life" of the unit (ibid.:19). Initially, they spent six months attending weekly discussions of cases, which were attended by nurses, social workers, doctors, and other professionals. Following this, they spent eight months on the unit, recording the unit's daily activities. They describe how they had to learn how to "fade quickly into the background or to be helpful in minor ways" (ibid.). There is an obvious contrast here with much (though not all) quantitative research, where the investigator seeks to structure and constrain the phenomenon of interest, whether by manipulating the independent variable in an experimental situation, or constraining the acceptable responses of the interviewee in a questionnaire study.

However, there is a big difference between observing that qualitative researchers have a preference for studying naturally occurring settings and claiming that this means that their research is "natural" (Silverman 1989, 1993; Hammersley 1992b). The notion that qualitative research (or indeed any research) is, or could be, natural raises several crucial problems. We considered the first of these—the idea that qualitative research can represent the world as it is—in the previous chapter. Any account of a setting, however rigorous, will always be "theory-impregnated." It is never possible to *reproduce* reality in our research reports. Reality will always be seen through a particular lens. There is a certain irony in simultaneous attempts to claim that all observation is theory-impregnated and that qualitative methods can access a natural world, as if the critique of observation were not equally applicable to all research (see Cicourel 1964).

The claim that qualitative research is "natural" presents a further problem, though. It is certainly true that most qualitative researchers seek to adopt a marginal role in the settings they study. Such marginality is seen as a way of reducing the reactive effect of the researcher's presence (Duffy 1987). It is an attempt to ensure that the phenomena observed by the researcher are unaffected by the researcher's presence, that people are undisturbed in their "natural habitats" (Becker 1970). Qualitative researchers' commitment to adopting a less intrusive role in the settings they study certainly contrasts with the approach of experimental and survey researchers, both of whom seek to create special settings for their research. However, the notion that qualitative researchers do not have an impact on the settings they study is patently false. Researchers may attempt to be passive and unobtrusive but their mere presence alters the setting in ways that may be significant. It would be naive to think otherwise. Indeed, as we shall argue in Chapter 4, one of the hallmarks of high-quality observational research is the researcher's attention to his or her impact upon the data generated. If this is true of observational studies, it is all the more true of interview studies, however little the researcher attempts to impose a structure on the interaction. Simply by being copresent, the researcher creates a context in which the things that informants say are influenced and constrained by their audience (i.e., the interviewer). Even, or perhaps especially, if the interviewer remains mute and expressionless, he or she will have an impact upon the talk that occurs within the interview. The implications of this feature of interview situations are discussed in more depth in Chapter 5.

A particular strength of qualitative methods is their ability to study human beings in the course of their everyday activities. The gains in validity are traded off against the ability of experimental social sciences to manipulate environments in ways that can allow a greater specificity. The qualitative researcher is more dependent on the search for natural experiments, settings that resemble, or differ from, each other in identifiable ways that are of theoretical interest. The researcher's intervention may be one of the tools of natural experimentation. What are its effects and what do they tell us about the setting? Early texts recommended a passivity that qualitative researchers are increasingly questioning (Cassell & Wax 1980; Emerson 1981; Hammersley & Atkinson 1995). The act of research makes most natural settings artificial.[2] We can, however, seek to learn about their natural state from our examination of what changes have identifiably occurred in its transformation by our involvement. Such reflection is, though, a means to the goal of learning about the world, rather than being turned inward as the romantics would have it, as a means to learning about the self.

MYTH NUMBER THREE: QUALITATIVE RESEARCH ALLOWS US TO CAPTURE THE UNDERSTANDINGS AND MEANINGS THAT MAKE PEOPLE BEHAVE AS THEY DO

This may be the most widespread myth of all. Again and again, in books and articles on qualitative research methods, we are told that the distinguishing feature of qualitative research is a commitment to uncovering the meanings that underlie people's behavior (Wiseman 1970; Lofland 1971;

Patton 1990; Duffy 1987; Merriam 1988; Habermann-Little 1991; Henwood & Pidgeon 1992; Oiler Boyd 1993a; Lindlof 1995). For such writers, qualitative research is all about understanding action in terms of the perspectives of those who are acting. By getting close to the people under study, by creating contexts in which people feel comfortable, we can persuade people to "tell it like it is."

It is not difficult to see why such a promise would be particularly attractive to people working in the health field. To take just the most obvious example, a great deal of patient behavior seems incomprehensible to practitioners and policymakers. Patients fail to complete courses of treatment, they behave in ways that they have been warned will have serious and even fatal consequences, they do not turn up for important tests when asked to do so, or they insist on consulting for demonstrably trivial problems. Numerous qualitative studies have been devoted to uncovering the meanings that lie behind these sorts of behaviors. This is presented as highly relevant research (Jensen 1989). If, the argument goes, we can understand what meanings underpin nonadherence to medical regimens we could, perhaps, find more effective ways of intervening that are sensitive to such meanings.

This enthusiasm for accessing the meanings underlying behavior is reflected in a number of the metaphors that pervade discussions of qualitative research. Qualitative research is seen as being able to "penetrate ... frames of meaning" (Bryman 1988:61) or to permit "penetration into their relational worlds" (Denzin 1970:133). It is described as "learning how informants interpret the world through which they move" (Agar 1980:90) and "stepping into the mind of another person" (McCracken 1988:9).

As with the two myths already discussed, the claim that qualitative research is concerned with penetrating meanings entails an implicit contrast with quantitative research, which is criticized for adopting methods that distance researchers from those they study and, as a result, rendering inaccessible the meanings that underpin behavior. Quantitative researchers are presented as adopting an "outsider perspective." This is compared with qualitative researchers' commitment to getting close to research participants through engagement with their everyday activities. Such involvement, whether through participant observation or qualitative interviewing, is seen as a means of achieving empathy with those who are being studied (Bryman 1988). Quantitative researchers are criticized for relying upon "remote, inferential materials" (Denzin & Lincoln 1994:5). Bryman sums up this supposed difference between qualitative and quantitative methods:

> The quantitative researcher adopts the posture of an outsider looking in on the social world. He or she applies a pre-ordained framework on the subjects being investigated and is involved as little as possible in that world. The posture is the analogue of the detached scientific observer. ...

Among qualitative researchers there is a strong urge to "get close" to the subjects being investigated—to be an insider. For qualitative researchers it is only by getting close to their subjects and becoming an insider that they can view the world as a participant in that setting. (1988:96)

As with the other two myths of qualitative research, this one is not without some foundation. Most qualitative researchers would agree that a distinctive feature of human behavior is that it is meaningful. This is one of the essential differences between the social and the natural worlds (Atkinson 1979). People are not automata who simply respond to stimuli. They are able to reflect upon and interpret both their own actions and the actions of people around them and such interpretations are significant influences upon their subsequent behavior. Indeed such interpretations may have a much greater impact on people's actions than the so-called objective facts of the situation.[3] In this respect, people are different from the phenomena that are studied by the natural scientist since, as far as we know, atoms, molecules, and so on do not interpret the environment in which they operate (Schutz 1962).

We accept, then, that one of the things that sets people apart from material objects is that they interpret their experiences. Such interpretations, and behaviors arising from them, will be informed by a wide range of ideas and theories that do not always map neatly onto medical theories. Many of these are shared in particular cultures and subcultures. It may well be that qualitative research allows us to identify some or all of the ideas that are current among individuals and groups. When asked about why they behave in one way rather than another, interviewees can be expected to display some of the ideas and theories that are current in the group(s) to which they belong. Likewise researchers who are observing the behavior of groups and individuals may well hear the explanations that individuals offer one another in the course of their ongoing activities.

Such data are certainly informative insofar as they can alert researchers and professionals to possible interpretations that would otherwise remain obscure. They allow us to identify the stock of knowledge, formulations, rhetorical strategies, and so on that are available to people in different contexts. However, it is a long way from this to the claim that such data allow us to explain a person's behavior. The problem of "other people's minds" is one of the oldest conundrums in the human sciences. How can we know what is going on in another person's head when we are not a telepathic species? Qualitative researchers have typically answered this by proposing an imaginative method. In the two most influential formulations—the idea of *verstehen* from the sociologist Max Weber (see Weber 1947: 87-115)) and that of "taking the role of the other" from the philosopher G. H. Mead (1934)—the process is conceived as a mental act on our part: If placed in the same situation as the other, how would I react? What would motivate *me*? However, our procedures for testing and verifying these claims are traditionally weak: as we noted in the previous chapter, they often come to little more than a claim to experiential authority. In recent years, there has been a shift in strategy to focus more on what people *do* and to use this as a more transparent and accountable basis for inductive reasoning. We can illustrate this with a brief discussion of interview data, which we shall develop in Chapter 5.

The problem here is that when interviewers ask someone to explain why they did what they did, they will receive an explanation that is designed to make the behavior in question understandable and reasonable to the particular person who asks. Technically, this is a "because of" account, "I did this because of the following reasons ..." This should not be confused with an "in order to" account, which might be offered in advance. "In order to" and "because of" explanations have no necessary relationship to each other and the relationship of either to whatever might have been in that person's mind at the time is indeterminate (Gould, Walker, Crane, & Lidz 1974). This is one sense in which the notion that qualitative research allows us to penetrate people's frames of reference to uncover the meanings that underpin their behaviors is mythical. We simply cannot argue that the explanations that people offer to us as researchers or to others in the settings under study allow us to grasp what was going on inside an individual's head as he or she decided to act in one way rather than another. At most we can claim that what we have elicited is an explanation that the interviewee or group member would expect to be treated as reasonable by the person to whom he or she is talking. This is an important point and we shall return to it several times in later chapters as we explore the implications.

However, this problem is not peculiar to interactions between interviewers and informants or even between researchers and the people that they study. It is an everyday problem for everyone. One of the miracles of society is the way in which we can manage the indeterminacy of meaning. We have evolved practical solutions to the problem of our lack of a telepathic faculty. An emerging agenda in qualitative research, associated particularly with an approach called "ethnomethodology," argues that we should focus on examining these practical solutions, which might then allow us to evaluate their efficiency and effectiveness (Emerson 1981; Hammersley 1992b; Silverman 1993). We will look more closely at this approach in Chapter 7.

However, we can illustrate some of the consequences of studying practices rather than eliciting meanings through Charles Bosk's book, *All God's Mistakes* (1992). Bosk carried out extensive firsthand observations among a team of genetic counselors employed in the clinical genetics center of a

Level III pediatric hospital. He joined the counselors' workgroup and attended preclinic conferences, observed counseling sessions, joined the counselors for postclinic conferences, interviewed a sample of parents, and was on call for emergency consultations with physicians in the newborn nursery and intensive care unit. From the data collected in these situations, Bosk constructed a detailed description of the genetic counselors' work, documenting its routines and operating procedures. He described his approach as follows:

> I think of clinical action in terms of situations—in particular those in which clinical action is problematic. Procedurally, I examine these situations to uncover what rhetoric, rationales, maxims, myths, data, and bottom lines physicians arm themselves with when they are recommending one course of action rather than another to patients, when they explain the unexpected, unwanted outcomes, and when they search for reasons to explain pain and suffering. (ibid.:4)

He listened to the counselors as they interacted with patients, with other physicians, and with one another. In the course of these interactions, the counselors routinely offered explanations of why they had behaved in particular ways. Bosk analyzed these explanations not as the motivations behind counselors' actions but as indicators of the professional ideologies and group norms that prevailed in the facility. He did not claim to have discovered why counselors did what they did. Rather he focused upon the ways in which the official clinic ideology of nondirectiveness and patient autonomy conflicted with other imperatives in the facility and the ways in which such tensions were dealt with in practice. In doing so, he was able to show how this ideology allowed the counselors to define their role very narrowly as that of technical experts whose sole responsibility was to pass on factual information. In turn this allowed the counselors to resist attempts to involve them and to distance themselves from any responsibility to engage with patients' distress or to advise parents about the most appropriate course of action.

CONCLUSION

In this chapter, we have examined three claims that are frequently made about the distinctiveness of qualitative research and found them to be seriously misleading. While all three myths incorporate some important truths, each presents distorted pictures of both qualitative and quantitative research. They exaggerate differences between these two traditions and downplay their common ground. Such polarization is particularly unhelpful in the health field, limiting as it does the potential for combining research methods in useful and creative ways.

We are not, however, arguing that there are *no* differences between qualitative and quantitative research. Indeed it is their very differences that create the greatest potential for positive and beneficial cooperation between these two traditions. Qualitative research is able to contribute to knowledge in ways that are different from and complementary to the contributions of quantitative research. This distinctive contribution is examined in the next chapter.

NOTES

1. "Waiting time" apparently comes with its own metric, the number of minutes between arrival and consultation, but it has actually been operationalized in the same way. It is simply that the measures of clock time are so universal that we do not usually notice that this has happened.

2. The observer in some large-scale and anonymous settings like crowds, theater audiences, or political rallies may be able to escape this to some extent. However we should not imagine that reflective observers in such settings directly reproduce the experience of participants. Their conscious reflection upon the experience immediately makes it an artificial one.

3. One of the most famous aphorisms in sociology is W. I. Thomas's observation, "If men define situations as real, they are real in their consequences." This is, however, usually cited without reference to its context, where Thomas makes it clear that he is not adopting a radically idealist position, merely noting that both "objective" and "subjective" features of situations can have real consequences. See the discussion in Murphy et al. (1998:46)

3

So What Is Different about Qualitative Research?

In the last two chapters we examined the popular claim that there is a fundamental divide between qualitative and quantitative research. We rejected the notion that qualitative and quantitative researchers are engaged in radically different enterprises. Consequently, we have no difficulty with the idea that studies using these different methods can, with integrity, be combined in the same research program. Where researchers share the goal of making truth claims, supported by rigorous and systematic data collection and analysis, intended to be useful to policymakers, practitioners, and service users, there is no reason why they should not coexist and collaborate. Qualitative and quantitative research into health and health care are complementary rather than competing strategies for data collection and analysis.

This does not mean, though, that there are no differences between qualitative and quantitative methods or that there are no grounds on which we might choose between them in relation to particular research questions. The needs of research users are not homogeneous and neither are the phenomena to be investigated. Some methods are more appropriate than others for particular investigations. This chapter discusses the kinds of research enterprise to which qualitative methods are particularly well suited and the ways in which they can be used alongside contributions from quantitative methods. Where the previous chapters stressed similarities, this chapter explores the real differences. When and why should research consumers think about commissioning qualitative research?

DESCRIPTION

Qualitative methods are particularly useful in providing rigorous descriptions of practice and the organizational contexts in which it occurs. Qualitative researchers develop skills in examining the routine, everyday, and taken-for-granted aspects of the settings they study. Observational methods, for example, allow researchers to provide detailed descriptions of what goes on in a hospital clinic, an in-patient floor, or a management meeting. These are likely to identify features of people's work and interactions that pass unnoticed by those actually involved because they have become so embedded in the background to their actions. However, an understanding of these features may be critical to achieving effective changes in working arrangements for the benefit of patients or the organization. They will have evolved over the life of the institution as practical solutions to the problems that its members encounter in their everyday work. Of course, as with any evolutionary process, some of these arrangements may well have ceased to serve their original purpose or even have become disabling for the institution. The point, however, is that any proposals for change that do not acknowledge, respect, and address the functionality of these practices, for those involved in them, are likely to provoke hostility, lack of cooperation, or active resistance. A manager or planner may still choose confrontation, but qualitative research can support a more thoughtful or subtle approach that goes with the grain of the institution rather than cutting across it.

It is precisely the thoroughly routine and unnoticed aspects of organizational life that tend to remain inaccessible to researchers using quantitative methods. To measure a phenomenon you first have to be made aware that it exists. By approaching a setting as an outsider, as someone who does not immediately understand why things are as they are, the qualitative researcher is less likely to assume that its current arrangements are inevitable and is more likely to question why things are one way rather than another. The description that they produce will not, of course, be the only possible description of the setting. As we saw in Chapter 1, any particular setting can be described in a number of different ways, reflecting what the observer takes to be relevant and, therefore, worth noting and reporting. As such, a researcher's description is a "representation" rather than a "reproduction" of the setting observed (Hammersley 1992e:23–24). A researcher, like any observer, can only proceed by paying attention to some aspects of the phenomenon that is being studied rather than to others. At the same time, the researcher can be expected to provide evidence to support the description that is produced through the research process. The usefulness of the representation presented to the commissioner will depend to a considerable extent on the quality of the original brief, and on the commissioner's appreciation that sometimes a report addressing an underlying issue that is discovered in the course of the research may be more useful than one so constrained by a tight brief that it ignores important data.

The potential value of detailed descriptions of the everyday life of health care settings is well illustrated in Guillemin and Holmstrom's (1986) study of newborn intensive care units, introduced in the last chapter. Unit staff clearly recognized, and were not unsympathetic to, the distress experienced by the parents of severely compromised newborn babies. However, they tended to see parents as traumatized and, therefore, as irrational and a potential threat to the well-being of their own infants. This view of parents as threats was used to justify various mechanisms through which the staff minimized parents' involvement in decision-making affecting their babies. The staff did not appear to recognize the ways in which the bureaucratic and clinical organization of the unit itself contributed to the parental distress, which was then subsequently interpreted as potentially threatening to the babies. As Guillemin and Holmstrom observed,

> It takes a tremendous effort for the [neonatal intensive care unit] staff to stand back from their work and ask this system-level question about lives they affect so deeply. (ibid.:196)

It is exactly this kind of standing back and asking questions that qualitative research does especially well. It can highlight significant dimensions of a phenomenon that would otherwise remain obscure.

Very often, as in the case of Guillemin and Holmstrom, qualitative methods will be the primary, if not the only, tools used in a study. However, their particular strength in providing detailed description of social processes and settings also points to the benefits of combining qualitative and quantitative methods in the same study. Most approaches to quantitative research require the researcher to identify the significant and important aspects of the phenomena of interest in advance of data collection. They also require the prior operationalization of those concepts that are judged to be significant, so that they can be measured reliably. Qualitative research can be used effectively as a precursor to such work, the rigorous description of naturally occurring settings and processes providing a basis for the clear specification of measures to be used in subsequent quantitative research.

If, for example, we want to compare the outcomes of two different "talking therapies" using a quantitative approach, it is vital that the two therapies first be rigorously defined. It is relatively easy to specify some external criteria. We could, for example, control for the length of sessions, the physical environment in which the counseling is carried out, the certification of

the counselor, the particular "school" to which the counselor claims affili-
ation, and so on. However, these features have an indeterminate relationship to what actually happens in a counseling session, which will always
be, to some extent, the joint product of the interaction between client and
counselor. Qualitative research, based on detailed observation of such interactions, can define homogeneous and commensurable categories of practice, which can then be used in an intervention study to compare their
relative effectiveness. Professional practice in this and many other health
areas is highly variable and even the best-defined protocols are subject to
modification in use.

The systematic and detailed description of what actually happens, rather
than what is supposed to happen, is a means of ensuring that the right
things are being counted in the most appropriate ways in quantitative
research.

PROCESS

A stress on the value of qualitative description should not be confused with
the claim, which is sometimes made, that qualitative research can only
describe and never explain. Indeed, careful, systematic, and rigorous description may, in itself, be explanatory. In particular, qualitative research can
help us to understand *how* a particular outcome arises. Qualitative research
is particularly well equipped to study the dynamic nature of settings and
behaviors. Longitudinal studies, for example, can fill in the gaps between
an intervention and its outcome. These studies focus on process rather than
impact. They can help to answer users' questions like, How does it work?
What is going on here? How did that come about? Why did that innovation work at a demonstration site but not here? Such questions are particularly important in health settings, given the high level of customization that
typically occurs when interventions are applied in particular contexts.

Carolyn Wiener's (2000) recent four-year study of assessment issues in
health care delivery in U.S. hospitals demonstrates how qualitative research
can be used to identify the processes that underlie observed outcomes.
Wiener examined quality assurance/improvement activities in U.S. hospitals. Her first step was to conduct a series of interviews with quality managers and coordinators in a variety of hospitals. This was followed by
participant observation[1] supplemented by interviews with key informants
in two very different hospitals. She observed meetings devoted to quality
assurance/improvement review, preparation for accreditation visits, nursing issues, administrative matters, the use of quality assurance/improve-
ment techniques, and redesign-planning and troubleshooting.

One of the initiatives Wiener studied was the attempt to apply to health care management the concepts and practices of "reengineering" and "work redesign," developed for the manufacturing and service sectors during the 1970s and 1980s. Redesign involved radical rethinking of work organization, directed to reducing costs while increasing customer satisfaction, quality, and market share. In one of the hospitals she observed, a firm of management consultants was hired to lead the redesign program.

Wiener describes several initiatives where much time, effort, and anxiety were expended in producing recommendations that subsequently failed at the implementation stage as a result of unanticipated factors. One such recommendation, for redistribution of work and cross training of personnel, proved particularly problematic. Here there was an attempt to achieve three goals. First, some work was to be reassigned to better-qualified staff. Second, some work was to be reassigned to those with less training who would be cheaper to employ. Third, there was an attempt to diversify the skills of individual staff members so that, for example, nurses would be trained to perform phlebotomies, record ECGs, and administer basic respiratory care. All these tasks had previously been the specialist preserve of other workers. The underlying objective was to achieve greater efficiency by matching tasks to skill levels among staff and reducing demarcation between staff, which was judged to be resulting in unnecessary idle time.

In practice, the redesign team attempted to achieve these goals through a combination of redundancies, reclassifications, collapsing job categories, hiring new workers, and retraining existing staff. The position of charge nurse/head nurse was replaced by that of "team leader." Such team leaders were assisted by two grades of "clinical partners." The first of these (Clinical Partner I) were the equivalent of licensed vocational nurses and the second (Clinical Partner II) were the equivalent of nurse attendants and patient support technicians. The latter were to combine the duties of housekeeping, delivering food trays, ordering and replenishing supplies, and transport.

Wiener identified a number of negative consequences that arose during this attempt at task rationalization. While both grades of clinical partner were pleased with the financial and occupational opportunities generated by the changes, registered nurses were angry about being required to relinquish the bulk of direct patient care to less-qualified staff. They argued that it was in the mundane care tasks that they were able to establish a relationship with patients and make important judgments about their health and functional status. They also complained about increased workload.

The impact on patients and other staff members proved even more problematic. For example, as part of the attempt to retrain generalist staff to carry out procedures that had previously been the preserve of specialist staff, most of the phlebotomists at the hospital had been dismissed or redeployed. Clinical partners were expected to take blood samples when necessary. Wiener describes, from her observations, how the problems generated by this transfer of responsibility soon became a recurrent theme at the meetings of the troubleshooting committee. The laboratory representative reported that she was getting frequent calls because staff were having difficulty in drawing blood. Given that she no longer had a team of phlebotomists available, she was unable to offer assistance and could only advise the callers to approach a doctor. In practice, attempts at flexible tasking led to the reallocation of tasks previously carried out by relatively cheap staff (phlebotomists) to more expensive grades (doctors). Moreover, difficulties in drawing blood led staff to use more expensive equipment since it could be more easily operated by relatively untrained and inexperienced people. Similar problems arose in relation to cuts in respiratory-therapy staff and the reallocation of their work.

Wiener describes the determination of the troubleshooting committee to persevere with the implementation of the redesign in spite of accumulating evidence of problems:

> As the committee struggled with these problems month after month, at times it seemed that their belief in redesign—sold to them at great economic and emotional cost—resembled the belief of Soviet revolutionaries that forced grain levies would foster a cooperative relationship between the peasantry and the state. (Wiener 2000:196)

Almost two years after beginning implementation, the hospital announced its conclusion: "'Redesign' has not delivered the desired impact on either quality of service or reduced cost" (ibid.:198). All the staff who had been reclassified as clinical partners reverted to their traditional roles.

A particular strength of Wiener's study is that she not only describes what happened but is also able to present detailed data on *how* it came to happen. Her prolonged immersion in the setting and careful documentation of the processes involved in the emergence, design, implementation, and eventual breakdown of the redesign initiative allowed her to identify some of the factors that turned a superficially rational and efficient organizational change into a costly, protracted, and disruptive failure. Among other things, she points to the lack of follow-through by the consultants who recommended the redesign, the lack of investment in the education of redeployed staff, a deficit in analytic skills among redeployed staff, and a lack of appropriate team leadership skills among the registered nurses.

This capacity for studying *process* suggests another way in which qualitative and quantitative research might be combined. Quantitative designs are particularly useful when it comes to examining relationships between inputs and outputs in health care. They can provide detailed and reliable outcome data, which, in principle at least, allow us to decide whether a particular intervention was worthwhile. However, such studies often lack explanatory power insofar as, while they can report the probability that intervention A will lead to outcome B, they are rarely able to tell us much about <u>how</u> A was transformed into B. Such outcome studies can usefully be combined with the kind of process studies that are possible using qualitative methods. This joint approach allows researchers to do two things, both of which are of great potential benefit to policymakers and planners. On the one hand, they can suggest the probability of a successful outcome arising from an intervention. On the other, they can provide important information about the factors that may have an impact between intervention and outcome, compromising or enhancing the success of the intervention under particular conditions. This is particularly helpful when it comes to the dissemination of successful interventions. Simple attempts to reproduce these at other sites often fail to match the achievements of the original. By specifying the environmental and organizational conditions that have contributed to that success, potential adopters can consider whether they can replicate these or find satisfactory alternatives.

FLEXIBILITY AND DISCOVERY

Wiener's study also provides an excellent illustration of another feature of qualitative research: its ability to deal with unanticipated factors or issues and to tell commissioners things that they did not expect to be relevant or to find out. Unlike most of their quantitative counterparts, qualitative investigators do not expect fully to specify their research design in advance of data collection. Qualitative study design is a flexible, iterative process. Wiener captures its essence in the introduction to her book:

> Unlike a project designed to test or verify a hypothesis, which requires strict adherence to a research design, with grounded theory data collection cannot be planned in advance (beyond initial forays into the field). The procedure followed by grounded theorists is called "theoretical sampling." The emerging theory points to the next steps—the sociologist does not know what they will be until guided by emerging gaps and/or research questions suggested by previous answers. (ibid.:12)

With such flexible designs, the qualitative researcher is able to respond to unanticipated opportunities that arise in the course of the research. For example, Wiener describes how a valuable source of data arose from a "combination of the accident and sagacity that marks unstructured research" (ibid.:10). Early in the research, while attending a conference sponsored by the Patient Care Assessment Council, an organization of quality assessment/improvement professionals, Wiener was invited to observe future meetings of the council. Discussions at these meetings proved to be a key source of data for the study, one that Wiener could not have anticipated at the outset. Similarly, toward the end of her lengthy research, Wiener uncovered the existence of an online network where quality assessment/improvement professionals discussed common problems and sought or offered advice and assistance to one another. She subscribed to the network and obtained important data that allowed her to assess the generalizability of her findings to other hospital settings where similar policies were being implemented.

This flexibility in research design reflects the emphasis that qualitative researchers place on discovery. Their methods offer opportunities to study social processes and social meanings through direct engagement with and immersion in the concrete reality of everyday settings (Hammersley 1992a). They approach settings or phenomena of interest assuming that they do not necessarily know in advance what is going to turn out to be important. Even where previous research suggests promising lines of investigation, the researcher holds lightly to these until their significance is confirmed empirically. In qualitative research, data coding and analysis are carried out alongside data collection. Preliminary analysis of data from early stages of the research guides ongoing decisions about strategies for future data. Such decisions may reflect a commitment to test out the scope of a generalization derived from one part of the research setting by considering whether it holds under different circumstances (Dingwall et al. 1998). Flexible designs leave scope for researchers to pursue significant leads and ideas as they emerge, particularly from early stages of the research. However, initial flexibility normally gives way to "progressive focusing" (Glaser & Strauss 1965a; Strauss & Corbin 1990). As the research progresses, the researcher narrows its focus and identifies the aspects or processes that will be given priority.

In practice, there is considerable variation in the extent to which the precise focus of a qualitative study is formulated in advance. In many cases, the constraints of obtaining funding, or gaining approval from institution-al review boards,[2] mean that researchers have to be more specific about what they plan to do than they might choose to be if driven solely by intellectual curiosity. Increasingly, also, researchers can draw on the findings of earlier studies in the same or related fields to specify, in advance, aspects of the phenomena they propose to study that will bear further investigation.

The flexibility of qualitative research designs offers particularly useful opportunities for uncovering aspects of situations that are discrepant with researchers' or practitioners' prior assumptions. This is illustrated by

Charles Bosk's study, *All God's Mistakes* (1992), introduced in Chapter 2. Bosk describes how his initial decision to study genetic counseling reflected a desire to be working at the medical frontier of dramatic advances in fetal and neonatal diagnosis and treatment. He assumed that this frontier was where genetic counselors would be operating. However, he soon discovered that this was not the case. When something dramatic did occur, professional colleagues from other specialties overshadowed the genetic counselors. He compares their role to that of extras in a movie. The "terrible ordinariness of genetic counseling as an everyday activity" (ibid.:xvii) became a focus for Bosk's investigation. He examined the counselors' attempt to preserve their own working agendas and professional autonomy in situations where they could not claim priority on the basis of treatment emergencies or life and death decisions. The flexibility of qualitative research design allowed Bosk to tailor his investigation to the characteristics of the setting that were uncovered in the early stages of the research.

Qualitative research's flexibility and orientation to discovery point to a further way in which it may profitably be combined with quantitative research. Hypotheses can be generated or needs identified that can then be incorporated into experimental or quasi-experimental designs. Randomized controlled trials are expensive to mount and often pose major ethical and practical problems. There is a very strong argument for ensuring that their design is as well informed as possible, so as to maximize both the inclusiveness and the appropriateness of the outcome measurements. For example, if we intend to investigate the impact of a new psychotropic drug on physical, psychological, and interactional functioning, there is a good case for carrying out some qualitative research at an early stage to identify and specify the full range of possible impacts. This discovery-oriented approach might also give clues to possible variations in response by age, gender, or ethnicity. Such data would inform the design of a subsequent trial, suggesting, for example, that the outcomes, costs, and benefits for each group might need to be analyzed separately.

The opportunities for effective combination of the flexibility of qualitative research and more traditional quantitative methods are illustrated in the study carried out by Kaplan and her colleagues on the impact of computerization upon the clinical laboratory services in a large teaching hospital (Kaplan 1986, 1987; Kaplan & Duchon 1988, 1989). They studied the introduction of a computer system, which replaced manual systems for managing testing, and the reporting of results to clinicians, in nine laboratories within the hospital. The researchers used a combination of qualitative and quantitative methods. The quantitative measures were designed to test preexisting theory about job characteristics and satisfaction and their relationship to reactions to the new computer system. These data were collected through questionnaires administered to laboratory staff seven months and approximately nineteen months after the installation of the new system. Qualitative data were gathered from a combination of interviews, observation, and open-ended questionnaire responses, carried out before, during, and after the installation. The qualitative and quantitative elements of the study were integrated insofar as the design of the questionnaires was informed by data from early qualitative interviews and, conversely, open-ended questions from the structured interviews were subjected to qualitative analysis.

The focus of the analysis was upon the similarities and differences among laboratory staff and across the nine laboratories and relationships between such variation and responses to the new computer systems. Kaplan's initial analysis of the qualitative data suggested that there were some substantial differences between different technologists and laboratories in their assessments of the impact of the new computer system. Some focused on increased workloads while others reported improvements in the communication of test results. However, these findings appeared directly to conflict with those from the quantitative data. Here the researchers examined the relationship between technologists' assessments of the impact of the new system and the standard measures of job characteristics and job satisfaction that had been incorporated into the questionnaires. They concluded that different reactions to the new computer systems were unrelated to differences between the computer technologists.

If the quantitative study had been carried out in isolation, the researchers would simply have concluded that differences in evaluation of the new system were unrelated to job characteristics. However, the qualitative study both raised doubts about the validity of these findings and suggested a means by which these doubts could be resolved. The flexible nature of the qualitative data collection had allowed the researcher to explore areas and follow up leads that had not been anticipated at the initial design stage. Revisiting the qualitative data, Kaplan was able to identify variation among the laboratory technicians, which was not reflected in the quantitative measures of job characteristics and job satisfaction used in the questionnaire study. These did not relate to the objective nature of the work but to the ways in which the technologists understood their jobs. Kaplan and Duchon described these differences:

> One group saw their jobs in terms of producing results reports, the other in terms of the laboratory bench work necessary to produce those results reports. The group who saw its job in terms of bench work was oriented towards the work of producing lab results, whereas the group who viewed its work in terms of reporting results was oriented towards the outcomes of the lab work: the members of this group saw themselves as providing a service. (1988:49)

This distinction became central to the subsequent analysis of both qualitative and quantitative data. In both cases, it was found that this difference in work orientation was indeed associated with different evaluations of the impact of the computer system on the operation of the services. Those who saw their work primarily in terms of producing results tended to view the new system as having a negative impact in terms of increasing workload and interfering with their established ways of working. The others, who defined their task in terms of providing a service through making results available, were more likely to offer favorable assessments of the new system. They saw it as a means of improving the service they offered to the rest of the hospital.

Contrary to the findings of the initial quantitative analysis, evaluation of the new system was found to be linked to technologists' orientation to their work. The standard job characteristic measures used in the questionnaire study to assess this orientation had proved insensitive to the variation in work orientation that existed in the particular local context. The consequence was a false negative result. By contrast, the flexible nature of the qualitative design, which allowed the researchers to identify those differences in job orientation that operated locally, rather than those extrapolated from general-level theories, proved effective in uncovering the links that did exist between job orientation and response to the new computer system. Moreover, the combination of qualitative and quantitative research meant that the tentative relationship between job orientation and evaluation of the new system found in the qualitative data could be checked out using the quantitative data set. This allowed the researchers to combine the flexibility of qualitative research with the enhanced generalizability typical of more quantitative approaches. Kaplan herself summed up the contribution of the qualitative arm of her study:

> It was not possible to design, in advance, a quantitative study that would have tested the right hypotheses, because appropriate hypotheses could not be known in advance. A qualitative approach enabled the researchers to see how individuals construed the information technology, their jobs and the interaction between the laboratory computer system and their jobs. Thus the researchers were able to generate productive hypotheses and theory. (Kaplan 1987:50)

CONTEXT AND HOLISM

The complex and contextual nature of all activity that involves human beings is a central issue for social and operational research. It is a particular issue in health research as the preoccupation with the placebo effect testifies. Any intervention, whether a drug, a treatment program, or an administrative reorganization, takes place in an organizational and relational context that, potentially at least, may have an impact upon its out-come. The same drug, program or reorganization, in a different context, may produce subtly and not-so-subtly different outcomes. Both qualitative and quantitative researchers are preoccupied with this interplay between activity and context. However, they engage with it in radically different ways.

In much quantitative research, with its dominant emphasis on isolating causal relationships between variables, contextual factors are typically assigned the status of potentially threatening contaminants to the integrity of a research design. The aim is to establish valid and reliable relationships, and, possibly, universal laws, which by definition hold irrespective of context. Such researchers are sensitive to the difficulties that are posed by the complexity of the social world and the ever-present risk of spurious correlations. Their aim is, as far as possible, to nullify the context and to try to eliminate the merely situational (Stake 1995). They look to physical and statistical controls as a way of identifying relationships that hold independently of context. Such controls are the means by which they pursue the holy grail of predictive theories based on isolation of cause and effect relationships between variables. Randomized controlled trials stand at the peak of this endeavor. Here, the aim is to control the effect of confounding variables, allowing the researcher to establish relationships that are expected to hold irrespective of context. Sophisticated multivariate analyses are a related attempt to deal with the complexity of relationships while, at the same time, holding other contextual factors constant. It is here, perhaps, that the contrasts between qualitative and quantitative research are most striking.

It is not that qualitative researchers are blind to the complexity of the social world. It is simply that we engage with it somewhat differently. Rather than trying to control complexity, we argue that it should be placed at the center of the researcher endeavor. This embrace of complexity can make qualitative research particularly helpful for managers and planners. Such people may yearn for simple remedies—and there are plenty of people who will peddle these for a price. In the real world, though, those who are trying to run or develop organizations know that they have to deal with complex systems that are involved in continuing and equally complex relationships with their environment. Most quantitative research inevitably strains toward simplification, limiting its ability to unpack the mixture of social, economic, political, and environmental factors that are at the heart of human action (Baum 1995). Quantitative work can "ride roughshod over the complexity of the social world" (Hammersley 1992d:32) and fail to engage with the way in which social variables are intrinsically more difficult to isolate and measure than those in the natural sciences (Silverman 1985). Mishler (1979) coined the term "context-stripping" to describe the shortcomings of such approaches.

A major problem arises when context-stripping is applied to research on the delivery of health care. The emphasis on controlling extraneous variables can have the consequence of ruling out of the analysis the very interactive effects that are typical of everyday health care settings. This creates major problems when it comes to generalizing from experimental situations to routine everyday practice. The factors that have been controlled as potentially confounding variables may turn out to have a crucial impact on the success of interventions in routine settings. Cochrane, a leading advocate of the randomized controlled trial (RCT), himself recognized this problem:

> Between the scientific measurements based on RCTs and the benefit measurements ... in the community, there is a gulf which has been much underestimated. ... Different strategies of management may be needed to reach levels of effectiveness comparable to those reached in RCTs. There is in addition the vast problem of the optimum use of personnel and materials in achieving those results. (1972:2)

Qualitative research seeks to bridge the gulf between the experimental situation and implementation in the community. By examining how interventions and initiatives interact with context, they can provide policymakers and practitioners with the basis for informed judgments about the likely impact of developments, which have been demonstrated unequivocally to be beneficial under controlled conditions, once they are implemented in the complex, and sometimes messy, contexts that are typical of everyday health care settings.

The importance of this interaction between intervention and context can be seen in a rather different qualitative study of the introduction of computer systems into clinical settings. Greatbatch and his colleagues investigated the impact of computerization on professional practice and interpersonal communication within health care consultations (Greatbatch, Luff, Heath, & Campion 1993; Greatbatch, Heath, Campion, & Luff 1995a; Greatbatch, Heath, Luff, & Campion 1995b). The study focused upon the installation and use of desktop computers in the offices of family physicians working in an inner-city area of northwest England. The new system allowed doctors to enter and retrieve details of patient illnesses and treatments and to issue printed prescriptions. Data entry and retrieval required the physician to follow a series of prompts, moving progressively through options generated by the computer. This system replaced previous arrangements under which records and prescriptions were handwritten by the physician.

Greatbatch and his colleagues video-recorded approximately 100 consultations before the introduction of the computer system and another 150 after its installation. The postinstallation recordings were collected at various time intervals to enable the researchers to detect any changes in the use and impact of the system as physicians became more familiar with its operation. The video data were analyzed using techniques derived from conversation analysis (Maynard 1989), which are discussed more fully in Chapter 7. These involve the repeated replaying and careful transcribing of recordings of naturally occurring interactions. Such transcription involves not only the content of what is said in the setting but also details of speech production such as pauses, overlapping talk, pitch, amplitude, and intonation. In the case of video recordings, details of gaze, gesture, posture, and so on are also included. The resulting transcripts serve as an index to the recordings in order to identify recurring patterns of action and interaction and look for tacit, taken-for-granted aspects of human conduct.

Using these techniques, Greatbatch and his colleagues were able to demonstrate that the introduction of computers had considerable impact upon the doctors' ability to record and retrieve information flexibly during the consultation. They identified a number of ways in which the computer system affected communication between doctor and patient. For example, they found that doctors frequently coordinated their interaction with patients with their use of the system. They delayed responses or paused in the middle of their talk until they had completed a sequence of keystrokes. Similarly, they found that patients were sensitive to the doctor's use of the computer, timing their utterances to coincide with the completion of particular computer-led activities by the doctor. Greatbatch and his colleagues concluded that the introduction of desktop computers undermined the physicians' abilities to carry out simultaneously the tasks of information retrieval and recording, and of displaying sensitivity to the patients' interactional needs. Even after two years, the computer system still compared unfavorably with paper records and written prescriptions in terms of interactional intrusiveness. Moreover, they were able to identify the particular characteristics of the computer system being used that contributed to these difficulties, suggesting ways in which future designs might be improved.

In this study, Greatbatch and his colleagues embraced the complexity of the contexts into which the new computer systems were to be introduced. They were mindful of a substantial body of research that shows that even where such computerized systems have been demonstrated to be technically and economically sound, they may not fulfill their potential to improve the efficiency and quality of health care delivery. Surveys of U.S. hospitals suggest that up to 50 percent of information systems fail, and that at least some of this failure is due to staff resistance and interference (Dowling 2001; Lyttinen 1987; Lyttinen & Hirschheim 1987). Rather than treating the context as a potential contaminant, Greatbatch and his colleagues focused on the interaction between the new technology and the social and relational environments into which it was introduced. As a result they identified the ways in which the use of computers affected, and was affected by, the interactional patterns, working practices, and relationships that are part of the characteristic messiness of everyday professional practice.

UNCOVERING THE INFORMAL ORGANIZATION

The various features of qualitative research that we have described—its concern for the everyday, its close attention to detail, its ability to deal with the unexpected—have also contributed to its capacity to address the issues that organizations would rather not know about, or have known. We have called these the informal life of the organization in order not to pass the implied judgments that terms like "deviance," "misconduct," or "stigmatized activity" might imply. The informal side of organizations is not more real or truer than the formal side (Dingwall & Strong 1985). It is just as much part of the organization as the legitimate, public, and authorized side that its members would like to present. Every organization, though, has its dark side and a full understanding of this is part of understanding what the institution is. A thoughtful leadership will want to know the bad news about its enterprise before this becomes a matter for public scandal, criminal investigation, or muck-raking journalism. Moreover, it will also want to understand how these unofficial arrangements arise and are sustained because they rarely reflect the actions of wicked, sinful, or corrupt individuals, as opposed to rational responses to everyday contingencies or to structural invitations to act in an unsanctioned fashion. The identification of the structural and interactional features of the environment that serve to hold inappropriate, ineffective, or dangerous behaviors in place is a task for which qualitative observational research studies are particularly well suited.

A good example of this is provided by Charles Bosk's work on how surgeons detect, categorize, and sanction medical error, *Forgive and Remember* (1979). Bosk observed two different surgical services at an elite U.S. medical institution affiliated with a major medical school:

> This involved following surgeons through their daily activities: I visited patients twice daily on rounds, drank coffee in the doctors' lounge during time-out periods, scrubbed in and assisted on operations when hands were

short, stood over bodies as they were pronounced dead, and stayed on call
at night and felt the rush of adrenalin a life-threatening emergency brings.
(ibid.:14)

In addition, Bosk studied attending physicians' written evaluations of
house staff and attended the faculty meetings at which decisions were made
to retain or terminate junior house staff in the training program.

Forgive and Remember provides a detailed analysis of how medical failure is defined, categorized, and responded to in the everyday lives of surgeons. Bosk points to some of the shortcomings of current systems of
accountability, particularly in terms of its their overreliance upon the individual consciences of surgeons and the lack of rigorous organizational
control that would open up the decisions and practices of individual surgeons to scrutiny and, where necessary, sanctions. One of the strengths of
Bosk's analysis is that he deals even-handedly with staff at all levels of the
organization under study.[3] While he concludes that changes in systems of
professional accountability and regulation are desirable, he resists the temptation to treat current practices as merely reflecting the self-interest, ava-
rice, or corruption of surgical staff. He makes understanding the cognitive
and social world of surgery central to his analysis. He shows how current
practices can be interpreted as a rational response to the contingencies,
uncertainties, and dilemmas that characterize surgical work (see also Pope
2002). In the introduction to his book, Bosk argues that any proposal for
change and improvement must be grounded in a thorough understanding
of the cognitive and social frameworks of current practice:

> Any programmatic change which intends to make professionals more ac-
> countable to clients must of necessity start with a complex phenomenologi-
> cal understanding of what currently passes for accountability and how it is
> achieved. Field research such as this informs policy by grounding it in a firm
> understanding of how participants construct their social worlds. It is only
> from this concrete understanding of the present, practical order that any
> changes in the existing interactional politics of social control can be negoti-
> ated. (ibid.:6)

It is just this sort of understanding that qualitative research is well-
equipped to supply.

CONCLUSION

The decision about whether to commission and use qualitative or quantitative methods, or a combination of both, is a pragmatic one. The overriding question should be, "What methods will provide answers to the

question at hand in the most effective and efficient manner?" In this chapter, we have suggested some of the circumstances where commissioners or users might choose to employ qualitative research either alone or in combination with quantitative techniques. There are no hard and fast rules here and, in most cases, the choice of method will involve a balancing of costs and benefits in the context of financial and other constraints. In Part II, we turn to consider how the various qualitative research technologies can contribute to the goal of building a sound evidence base for the delivery of health care.

NOTES

1. See Chapter 4 for a detailed discussion of the method of participant observation.

2. This is more fully discussed in Chapter 8.

3. See our discussion of "fair dealing" in Chapter 9.

II

The Practice of
Qualitative Research

4

Observation, Interaction Analysis, and Documents

Qualitative research is often discussed as if it were something new and revolutionary. In fact, of course, it has been around as long as human beings have inquired into the nature of the world about them and their relations to it and to each other. As a distinguished anthropologist once remarked, in an after-dinner speech, "There really are only two ways of getting information about social life: hanging out and asking questions." That statement, at least, will have been true throughout the history of our species. Interview research, whether qualitative or quantitative, is merely a recent way of "asking questions," while most observational research is a more or less elaborated way of "hanging out." The family of "hanging out" methods has, however, now been extended beyond simple observation. With the advent of audio and video recording, observation has been developed into interaction analysis, using the ability to preserve and replay situations in ways that recover more detail than traditional ear, eye, and hand methods can register. Anthropologists, of course, deal mainly with preliterate societies. Modern health care systems are found in literate societies, or the literate sectors of more traditional societies. The copious amounts of documentation they generate make an additional source of data available: "reading the papers," using documentary evidence as a means of observing participants working to create "official representations" of their activities.

This chapter focuses on these "hanging out" methods, although the language of after-dinner speeches may not do justice to the disciplined process of inquiry that is actually involved, as we have suggested in earlier chapters. More formally, we shall look at those methods that involve direct and systematic observation of the social processes involved in modern health care. Membership in this family is conferred by the use of "given" data.

It is important to understand that observational data are never a simple copy of reality, of the naturally occurring life of the institution being studied that exists prior to, and independently of, the intervention of the observer. However, such data are the result of a single transformation by the researcher in rendering reality into material suitable for analysis. Interview data, by contrast, involve at least two transformations, first by the interviewer who chooses the questions to ask and second by the respondent who restructures their original experience in the course of replying. In some cases, there may even be a third transformation if the researcher also proposes what the possible answers might be.

It is the minimization of this "chain of transformation" that explains why qualitative researchers tend to treat observational methods as their "gold standard" so that data derived from them carry more credibility than those derived from interviews. Researchers know that the only transformative intervention is their own. Part of the task that will then face them, of course, is to produce reports that will allow readers to assess the nature of that intervention and its implications for the correspondence between the data and the original reality. What has the researcher introduced between the observed events and the published analysis? As we saw in Chapter 1, this intervention has sometimes led to calls for the dissolution of the distinction between scientific reports and other forms of writing. While we rejected that argument, it is nevertheless clear that fair dealing between researcher and research user requires some declaration of interests, motives, and standpoints and some consideration of the extent to which these may have colored the process of data collection, and later analysis. This point is taken up again in Chapter 9.

Traditionally, anthropology and sociology relied on the fieldwork skills of observers and their ability to reproduce the fleeting and ephemeral character of events in their fieldnotes. The first section of the chapter examines this process. More recently, social scientists have increasingly used the technological aids of audio and video recording to freeze these moments so that they can be relived and reexamined in rather different ways. We shall discuss some of the implications of this shift. Finally, we shall look at the study of organizational documents. By these, we mean an organization's official representations of its own activities in records, reports, promotional materials and the like, as opposed to elicited documents like diaries or visualizations, which we shall discuss in the next chapter. These exist somewhere between the worlds of observation and of interviewing. They are like observation in the sense that they are "given" data. They are like interviews in the sense that they are artful reconstructions of the events that they describe, although, unlike interviews, they also form part of these events. They help us to understand how the organization represents itself to itself and to its environment. Modern health care generates vast record systems. If we look at these in ways that are different from those traditionally adopted by the social epidemiologist or statistician, what can they tell us?

OBSERVATION

> In its most inclusive sense, field research is simply research conducted in natural social settings, in the actual contexts in which people pursue their daily lives. The fieldworker ventures into the worlds of others in order to learn firsthand how they live, how they talk and behave, what captivates and distresses them. Whether it is the classic anthropologist trekking across the world to live with some remote tribe, the urban ethnographer moving into some hidden segment of the modern city, the participant observer sharing in and observing the lifeways of a local community or joining the rush-hour commute to study the lifeworlds of modern bureaucrats, the fieldworker's first commitment is to enter the ongoing worlds of other people to encounter their activities and concerns firsthand and close up. (Emerson 2001:1)

Emerson prefers the term "field research" for what others would more commonly call "participant observation," the study of social life by direct immersion in its everyday processes. Nevertheless, his description nicely captures the range of settings in which this craft may be practiced. The participant observer in a contemporary clinic is engaged in essentially the same activity as the anthropologist in the remote Highlands of New Guinea or the urban ethnographer hanging out with drug dealers and pimps on some inner-city street corner. In each case the goal is similar: to collect data from the direct observation and recording of talk and behavior that will allow the observer to specify the rules, conventions, or principles that organize these social worlds.

We will examine the inferential processes involved in the movement from recording to specification in Chapter 7. For the moment, it is enough to note that this is a key distinction between social science and muckraking journalism or fiction. The social scientist is less concerned with the exotic or the scandalous than in understanding what each can tell us about the mundane organization of everyday social life. When Bosk (1979), for example, studied the review conferences that followed possible cases of surgical error, his focus was less on exposing incompetent surgeons than on explaining how a system that was designed to identify and eliminate incompetence failed to do so. In the process, he shows that simple remedies would not capture the complexity of the problem, namely, the very real difficulty in separating surgical error from the inevitable challenges posed by the uncertain material that the surgeon is working on. Real human organs are not laid out in the neat shapes of anatomy textbooks. Real tissues vary in fragility and geometry, making standardized interventions difficult or impossible to achieve. When it is hard to separate the incompetent from the unlucky, surgeons have genuine difficulty in making the clean judgments about each other's skills that patient advocates increasingly demand.

The value of work like this to patients, professionals, and health care managers lies in its demonstration that the task of improving surgical practice and minimizing errors will require quite a sophisticated understanding of the intersection of the cultures and structures of a number of occupational groups, and the work settings in which they interact. However, it also reminds us that perfect outcomes cannot be guaranteed because of the inherent unpredictability of the intersection between surgical technologies and human bodies. A surgeon can perform the right operation with a high degree of professional skill and still have the patient die or suffer an adverse outcome. There may then also be an issue of expectations: If a hospital uses press advertising declaring, "It takes three to have a healthy baby—mom, dad and your obstetrician on staff at (Name) General Hospital," it is not surprising that any parent who has a less than healthy baby may wonder what part the obstetrician has played in that outcome.

PARTICIPATION AND OBSERVATION

What does participant observation look like? As the label suggests, it typically has two elements—participation and observation. These are often seen as points on a continuum (Gold 1969) but it may be better to acknowledge that all research is likely to involve both elements to a greater or lesser extent at different times. Complete observation, where the researcher is invisible and entirely passive, is relatively uncommon in qualitative research but does occur. In Miller's (1997) study of brief therapy, for example, he sat alongside consulting therapists behind a one-way mirror observing the interaction between the working therapists and the clients. The consulting therapists would telephone their colleagues in the working room from time to time and make suggestions about the direction that the interview was taking so clients were aware of the people behind the mirror. In this sense, even apparently invisible people were participants in the therapeutic encounter. Miller was also, clearly, a participant in the activities behind the mirror as the consulting therapists discussed the scene they were watching and possible interventions. However, his presence and note-taking was not continuously visible to clients.

By contrast, Bosk (1992) describes his direct observation of genetic counseling sessions, at the invitation of the counselors and introduced to clients as a sociologist working with the team. He discusses the way in which this effectively made him a participant, as what he came to call a "witness" to the counselors' practice in trying to deal both ethically and legally with highly sensitive issues. The counselors' enthusiasm for his study made him more of a participant than had been the case in his earlier (Bosk 1979) study of surgery:

> I was ornamental, decorative, extraneous, and dispensable. If I kept out of the way, if I was marginally helpful, if I filled rare down-time with interesting talk, whatever I wrote later was my own business. ... I was expected to contribute nothing fundamental to the ongoing life of the group. When I did help, when I opened packages, passed supplies or was simply an extra pair of hands, it was a welcome surprise to the surgeons. (Bosk 1992:7–8)

The actual balance between participation and observation is never entirely within the control of the fieldworker. The craft of field research lies in knowing when to lean in one direction and when in another and to be clear whether this is a matter of choice or contingency.

The sort of participant observation most typically carried out in health care settings is likely to involve some form of "person shadowing," where the fieldworker attaches him- or herself to members of the organization for periods of time and tracks them through their routine work. This may be complemented by "place shadowing," where the fieldworker remains in a particular location and watches organization members pass through it. When we write about "organization members" here, we are not necessarily excluding patients or clients—while they are in contact with the health system, it is often useful to think of them as members of that system. Millman's description of her approach to studying surgeons working in three U.S. hospitals catches the essence of what is involved:

> My usual method in this research was to attach myself for a time to a particular physician (most often a resident, but frequently a department chief or an attending doctor) and to follow that individual throughout his or her daily rounds of the hospital. For example, on the days I followed a surgical resident or team of residents I would arrive at the hospital at six-thirty in the morning, change into a surgical dress and a laboratory coat, and accompany my residents first on morning rounds, then to breakfast, and afterward into the operating room where they would spend a large part of the day. During surgery I usually stationed myself next to the anesthesiologist, by the patient's shoulders, so that I could watch the operation and listen to the conversations of the surgeons and staff as they worked. Between operations I joined the residents and nurses in the operating room (OR) staff lounge so that I could learn what was happening in other operating suites. Since I was free to wander, I could then circulate to whatever operating rooms were the scenes of

interesting incidents on any particular day. After surgery, I joined the residents
as they made afternoon rounds throughout the wards, performed "work-up"
examinations and attended various staff meetings. On patient rounds, when
I was introduced at all, it was simply as "Dr Millman" and "one of the team."
I ate lunch and dinner with the residents I followed. Occasionally, when the
resident I followed was on night call, I, too, stayed in the hospital through
the night. (1976:14)

We have quoted this at some length because it makes a number of points.
It shows a fieldworker who is carrying out both people shadowing (residents, chiefs, or attendings) and place shadowing (staff lounge). Both of
these activities imply decisions about whom or what we study within the
setting at any particular time. (The issues of sampling will be discussed in
more detail in Chapter 6.) It also conveys something of the intensity of fieldwork—notice the way in which Millman writes about "*my* residents." To
understand surgery, you need to be wherever surgeons are at whatever
times they are doing their work. Much health care is not confined to office
hours and there are quite significant differences, in hospital work, for example, depending upon whether you are observing a service during the
daytime or at nights and weekends (see Zerubavel 1979). The kind of commitment involved becomes increasingly difficult to combine with academic
careers and family lives, so that research commissioners often need to make
a hard choice between expensive buyouts of experienced investigators or
accepting that work will be done by relatively junior people, with fewer
competing claims on their time, and hoping that adequate supervision will
be available for them. It is also important to see that adequate downtime
is built into the research timetable, where researchers can reflect on what
they are observing and, if necessary, correct their strategy and tactics. The
extract also shows the strategies that Millman adopted to become unobtrusive—wearing surgical greens and a white coat, sharing the routine of the
resident's life, finding a place to stand in the OR that allowed her to moni-
tor communication and action without obstructing the operating surgeon.
During ward rounds, she merges into the team and consciously minimizes
her presence while work is being done.[1]

This passage emphasizes her role as an observer. However, it is also clear
that much of her data comes from informal conversations, as well as the
formal interviews that she carried out with some of the most powerful
actors in these hospitals. Although participant observers tend to emphasize the given nature of their data, their work often relies on material that
they have solicited or provoked from participants. These are sometimes
called "natural interviews," that is, conversations that take place with the
objective of eliciting data. Occasionally, although it can be a risky strategy,
a fieldworker may try to discover more about a setting by deliberately
breaching one or more of its everyday conventions. In his work on child

protection (Dingwall et al. 1983), for example, Dingwall became interested in understanding the basis of social workers' adherence to professional standards in the absence of managerial surveillance. One particularly trusted informant was dealing with a pregnant teenager on her caseload and considering how to tell an absent and disengaged parent about her decision to give consent to an abortion without running the risk of prompting parental intervention. Dingwall pointed out that she had the option of writing such a letter, placing a copy in the file, and destroying the original, blaming nonreceipt on the postal service if subsequently challenged by the parent. Although this is not discussed in the book, he then used her reaction to this suggestion as a means of exploring her sense of professionally or organizationally correct behavior and subsequently employed the episode as a vignette in natural interviews with other social workers to determine whether her temptation and rejection would be recognizable to them.

It is essential that data collection and analysis acknowledge the difference between what is overheard or witnessed and what is generated by the direct intervention of the fieldworker. We shall look at this issue more closely when we discuss fieldnotes, in the next section, and analysis, in Chapter 7.

RECORDING DATA

If the degree of participation is a matter of some negotiation, observation is the inescapable core of the method. Fieldworkers have something of the Recording Angel about them. Their objective is to make as an accurate a record as possible of the events that go on around them, and of their own responses to these. Each of these elements needs some further discussion.

Although fieldnotes are the foundation of observational research, it is only recently that people have begun to discuss them explicitly. This is partly because observational methods were often passed on in a craftlike fashion from master to apprentices. Indeed, it is still striking how much the acknowledgments of qualitative studies trace a narrow line of descent to a handful of scholars working in the 1950s and 1960s. With the expansion of training to supply a higher level of societal demand for social researchers, other means of dissemination have become necessary. An oral tradition has begun to be inscribed (Sanjek 1990; Emerson, Fretz, & Shaw 1995).

Fieldnotes have tended to be intensely personal documents. There are several reasons for this. One, clearly, is the confidentiality of the people and situations described in them. Participant observers often have access to material that is very sensitive and potentially damaging to individuals and organizations. By the time that this appears in print, it has been through a process of editing that is intended to disguise its sources, in ways that do not compromise the analytic points made by the data that are presented. However, the data cannot begin like that. In the field, notes name real people, use their actual words so far as possible, and specify dates, times and places. Second, the acknowledgment that the credibility of participant observation data turns to some degree on observers' self-analyses, to determine what effects they are having on other participants in a setting and to specify just what knowledge they are using to identify what might be significant, means that there is also a good deal of sensitive data about observers as well. A particularly extreme example of this is the anonymous account by "Cesara" (1982), a Canadian anthropologist. Her book explored, from the notes that she had made in the field, the tensions in her relationship with her husband back home and the extent to which her access to data had rested on her sexual relationships with men in the African community that she was studying. Involvements of this kind seem to be unusual, and are certainly not to be recommended as ethical models, but are only a matter of degree. Most fieldnotes contain material about the observer's reactions to the fieldwork site and the other people in it that they would not wish others to access in a raw form. The anthropological community was deeply riven in the 1960s, for example, by controversy over the publication of the private field diaries written during fieldwork in Melanesia between 1914 and 1918 by one of its founders and heroes, Bronislaw Malinowski (1967), and the question of whether comments about his local informants that had never been intended for publication characterized him as a racist. Finally, and quite practically, fieldnotes are often not very intelligible to other readers in the sense that they are written as an *aide-memoire* that will allow the researcher to reconstruct events and conversations from memory at a later date. The notes need to be "filled in" to be fully usable.

To the extent that we can generalize, however, contemporary "best practice" would probably recognize three features as crucial to the accuracy of data. First is the desirability of making notes at the time that observations are being made. Traditionally, notes were often made at some distance from the event. Researchers would go into bathrooms, find empty corners of buildings, or slip out during lunch breaks. They would then seek to recall key information and jot down as full a version as was practicable under these constraints. While this practice is still important, and essential in some environments, there is now greater acknowledgment that notes can be taken openly, that this gives a more accurate rendering of the talk, actions, and settings being captured in them, and that it may be marginally more ethical, in the sense that other participants have a continuing reminder that they are being observed and an opportunity to go "off the record."

Second is a degree of "behaviorization" of the first recordings. Jackson (1990:7) notes the regret of anthropologists whom she interviewed about their notes that they had not given more attention to getting the exact words used by the people being studied rather than describing their own impressions of the scene. This partly reflects the competition from audio and video recordings, discussed later in this chapter, and partly a recognition that the directly quoted voices of informants constitute evidence in a way that the observer's redescriptions and use of indirect speech do not. Although there are many issues about the basis on which particular quotations are selected for reproduction and discussion, which we shall look at in Chapter 7, behaviorization minimizes the chain of transformation.

Third, this shift has tended to formalize an injunction that was sometimes more honored in the breach than in the observance, namely, to ensure that the processing of field observations carefully tracked the status of each entry. Although we often talk glibly about fieldnotes, it is important to recognize that these normally involve three rather different kinds of text. They begin with the "jottings" that are made in the setting, which may be more or less detailed depending upon the extent to which they are made as things happen or in the bathroom afterward. Observers often develop private shorthands for this. These are then "written up" in the sense that the researcher produces a fair text, as soon as practicable after the original jotting, which reviews and consolidates the originals and expands on the shorthand. This process can also involve further filling in from memory of details that did not form part of the original jotting but that are recalled under the stimulus of the review. When researchers proceed to analysis, this is generally the version on which that stage is based. Notes of this kind are also more easily usable by colleagues in larger scale studies that involve sharing of data. Alongside this text can be found a parallel text, sometimes interpolated and sometimes kept in a separate journal, which records the researcher's reflections. As we have noted, these may be personal but they are also likely to be intellectual. The researcher records emerging hypotheses, apparent patterns of behavior, or echoes of previous research reports. These link into emerging ideas about the research strategy: Should the fieldworker be looking to sample particular kinds of event? Could there be counterexamples somewhere else? Is this an emerging generalization and how would it relate to others?

As we have already stressed, the fieldnote cannot be claimed to be a literal representation of the setting to which it relates. Its construction involves a considerable degree of intervention by the observer. The decision to record some things rather than others is an intervention. The process of transforming jottings into text is an intervention. Ultimately, the selection of extracts from the text for incorporation in the research report will also be an intervention. At the same time, the fieldnote is still disciplined by the events that it relates to, particularly if the observer is clearly marking the differences between those events or interactions that they have overheard or witnessed and those that they have prompted, in the form of natural interviews or interventions. Only the former are "given" data, while the others must be treated as closer kin to the interviews discussed in the next chapter.

In principle, the note should be recognizable to the participants. This is not to say that they have to endorse it. In a recent piece of fieldwork in a genetics research laboratory, for example, Dingwall made particular note of the different styles of lab coat favored by different members of the team. As an experiment, the principal investigator in the lab was reading his notes after they had been written up and found this particularly puzzling. Why was he wasting time on such trivia? In fact, as Dingwall explained, this was not, from his point of view, a trivial observation. He was referring back to research that had been done in the 1950s by Julius Roth (1957), observing sanatoria for tuberculosis patients. Roth had noticed the way in which protective clothing was a symbolic marker of status boundaries in these institutions. Essentially, the higher the status of a person, the less likely he or she was to wear a mask or gown. One way to identify where a person was located in the institutional hierarchy was to look at what they wore on the wards. Dingwall had drawn inspiration from this in the early 1970s during his own Ph.D. research on public health nurses. The public health department had just abolished the nurses' uniforms and substituted vouchers allowing them to buy "civilian" clothing instead. However, these vouchers could only be exchanged at rather conservative department stores, allowing the public health department to continue control of the image presented by its staff. When going into the unfamiliar setting of the laboratory, and being instructed in the health and safety requirements for protective clothing, Dingwall was immediately alert to the possibility that there might be some organizational significance to this, particularly when he picked up some lab gossip about one of the postdocs who had recently been reprimanded for persistent breaches of these requirements. None of this, of course, was evident in the fieldnote.

This experience underlines some of the earlier points about the personal nature of fieldnotes. Dingwall knew why he was recording these observations and did not even think them worthy of particular comment in a parallel text. When he returned to the data for analysis, he would expect to see the significance of these notes without any other flagging. Another researcher with a different intellectual biography would not necessarily pick up on this. It also illustrates the different orientations of participants and observers. Even after the observation was explained, the scientist involved had difficulty in seeing the connections between this set of observations over a fifty-year period and the way in which they meant that a person's decision to wear a distinctive style of lab coat might signify more than an expression of their taste. Finally, it brings out the selection decisions of the fieldworker. Dingwall noted the clothing details because he knew from literature and prior experience that they might come to have importance. These were events that happened, a reality that constrained his observations. Nevertheless, it was his choice to notice and record them.

These selection decisions may require more explication. In the classic accounts of participant observation, the researcher is often made to sound like a piece of clay that is ready to absorb whatever imprint the field places on him or her. More recently, there is a tendency to present the researcher as a latter-day Procrustes, forcing the field into the preconceived political or normative frames that he or she has brought to it. The actual practice of fieldwork is somewhere in between. On the one hand, the researcher is trying to be open to the intrinsic nature of the field setting. On the other, he or she inevitably brings a range of scientific knowledge and personal experience that structure that openness. Fieldwork is not an aimless process.

The looseness of classic accounts of observational research practice partly reflects the shallow history of formal methodological writing and the limited scale of institutionalized qualitative research until the 1960s. The contrast with quantitative social sciences should not be overstated here (Platt 1996). Much of the impetus toward the production of both quantitative and qualitative methodological texts arose from the huge expansion in higher education after World War II. New strategies for teaching and learning were needed to deal with this mass market. In qualitative research, for example, no U.S. textbook seems to have been published between Vivien Palmer's *Field Studies in Sociology* (1928) and Buford Junker's *Field Work* (1960). When influential texts like Glaser and Strauss's (1967) *The Discovery of Grounded Theory* portrayed each fieldworker as an innovator, this was highly likely to be true. The world was full of places where no ethnographer had gone before and where there were few models or conceptual frameworks that might serve as points of orientation. Several decades later, it is much less likely that a researcher will be dealing with a site that is entirely novel, except in the trivial sense that one cannot step in the same river twice. Strauss (Strauss & Corbin 1990) subsequently came to accept that successful observational work drew heavily on the intellectual capital of the fieldworker, although Glaser (1992) continued to hold the original position (see Melia 1997).

An overemphasis on innovation, and a neglect of the need to assemble relevant ideas and concepts from previous studies, obstructs the development of models and generalizations that may have wider value to research users. It may also unduly prolong fieldwork by slowing the process of focusing on key issues. Dingwall's prior reading and previous experience, for example, led him to make systematic notes on the wearing of lab coats from the first day in the field. The period of fieldwork happened to be too short to determine whether this had any real significance but sufficient data would rapidly have been assembled. A more general example of this process of prior sensitization may relate to the role played by documents in modern organizations. There is such abundant evidence of the important role played by, material or electronic, texts in these environments that anybody planning to study a doctor's office, a clinic, or a hospital will almost certainly need to design a research strategy that makes reference to these artifacts. Who writes them? Who reads them? When and for what purposes? (We shall look at the issues around documents in more detail later in this chapter.)

AUDIO AND VIDEO RECORDING

As we noted above, the movement toward more behaviorized note-taking in observation studies is partly a response to the challenges of new technologies, particularly the emergence of lightweight audio and video recording equipment. These are sometimes claimed to transcend the process of transformation between reality and data by allowing analysts and readers unmediated access to the original events. In practice, it is more accurate to say that they can reduce the scope of transformation rather than eliminating it.

The God's eye camera and the perfect transcript do not exist. We remain dependent on where equipment is placed, what it can capture, and how that selection is reduced to a format capable of being analyzed and communicated. We may be able to reduce our reliance on the observer's memory for the details of talk or behavior and to acquire new information as a result of the ability to retain and review the events that have been recorded. If challenged on the accuracy of our renderings, we can replay the recording as a check on the transcript and on the analyst's interpretations of what they have heard or seen. However, just as the observer decides who to shadow and where to sit, recording devices can only capture what happens within their range and capacity. Sometimes this can be close to the idealization of the complete observer, like Miller (1997) sitting behind the one-way mirror in brief therapy. A researcher interested in traffic flows in a hospital reception area, for example, might use recordings from a surveillance camera installed for security purposes. More commonly, equipment is installed for specific research purposes and decisions are made about where it should be located, where it should be directed, who should focus or track it, and so on. Even if we use multiple cameras, decisions remain about which one to look at and how to choose between the versions offered.

Audio recording cannot capture movements and nonverbal communications, although this is a less serious problem than many critics claim unless one is looking at settings where the coordination of talk and movement is a core task, like operating rooms or physical therapy suites. The limitation can often be remedied by supplementing audio recording with some direct observation. Both video and audio data are difficult to incorporate into published reports, partly because of the technical editorial work needed to preserve confidentiality and partly because of the continued dominance of printed text. Since it is difficult to deliver copies of recordings alongside the text, some form of notational system is required to convert these sources into print, raising its own set of issues about what can be preserved and what is lost in the transformation (Graffam Walker 1986). The privileging of print also means that there is a tendency to imagine that the transcript is the primary data rather than the original recording. In fact, it is the recording that is the "given" data, not the transcript.

Recording, whether audio or video, is not a panacea. Its static nature means that it is best suited to place shadowing, where activities are going on in reasonably predictable ways and where prior decisions can be made about when and where to point cameras and fix microphones. Satisfactory recording often requires some prior observational work of a quite traditional nature to help refine the research strategy. We might envision a future of cyborg-researchers, where ethnographers could wear a camera that tracks and records their eye movements and lays down a sound recording that captures the interaction around them. However, the result could well be data overload, where so much information is produced without filtration by the fieldworker's stock of intellectual capital that it cannot be made to yield any useful or meaningful results. This can already be a problem with video recordings unless considerable prior thought has been given to the research questions that they are being used to address.

Nevertheless, recording has made an important contribution to the way in which some social processes in health care are understood, particularly because of the way in which the possibility of replaying recordings allows researchers to look much more closely at what is happening when people are interacting with each other and with their material environment. Replays also allow data to be shared more easily with other researchers and for analysis to be scrutinized more closely by peers.

INTERACTION ANALYSIS

The capacity of audio and video recording to retain data in forms that permit endless action replays has led to the development of new kinds of analytic procedures that have challenged some of the established findings of traditional modes of qualitative research, particularly about the nature of practitioner/patient interaction. Essentially, these replace the researcher's use of imaginative understanding or *verstehen* (see Chapter 2), with a requirement that proposed interpretations be supportable by reference to the actual talk and behavior of the people being studied. Rather than inferring the meaning of some utterance by imaginatively placing herself or himself in the position of the producer and trying to reconstruct what must have been in that person's mind to say such a thing, the researcher looks at what the recipient or recipients of the utterance do in response. To say that a physician asks a patient a question, for example, is not a matter of grammar or syntax or of "taking the role" of the physician. It is a claim that rests on the patient treating the utterance as a question and producing a response or, alternatively, indicating that it has been heard as a question but is not going to be treated as such. If neither of these responses is available, the researcher may inquire how an apparent question was not recognized or acknowledged as such or whether there is any evidence of deliberate or neglectful inattention. However, all these possible interpretations must be related back to the sequence of interaction within which the proposed question and answer/nonanswer are embedded. We shall look at the process of analysis more closely in Chapter 7.

For the moment, however, we can just note some of the practical uses to which work using these new procedures could be put: increasing the effectiveness of advice and information-giving [e.g., Heritage and Sefi (1992) on public health nurses; Silverman (1997) on HIV counseling; Pilnick (1999) on hospital pharmacists], delivering bad news to patients [e.g., Maynard (1991a, 1991b; 1992) on informing parents about disabilities in their child], rationalizing prescribing (Mangione-Smith et al. 2003) and improving communication between callers and call-takers for 911 services [e.g., Garcia & Parmer (1999) on delayed response due to incorrect classification]. There is also an emerging body of work, generally based on video recordings, dealing with the interaction between people and equipment [e.g., Greatbatch et al. (1995a, 1995b) on computer use in primary care consultations; Pilnick & Hindmarsh (1999) on anesthetic induction].

DOCUMENTS

As we noted at the beginning of this chapter, organizational documents lie somewhere between observational data and the interview data that we will discuss in the next chapter. To anticipate, they have some of the problems of interviews in being used as evidence of what people and organizations actually do. However, they can be valuable evidence about what people and organizations would like to be thought to be doing. By analyzing documents in this fashion, we may be able to learn many useful things about the ways in which work is represented and about the possible relationship between representations and performance. Some of the results of such analyses have considerable implications for the validity and reliability of many conventional measures of performance and for the interpretation of data from certain types of quantitative research study in health care. This section will focus on three particular topics: the social construction of organizational statistics, the internal and external representation of organizations, and the interaction between work and documents.

THE SOCIAL CONSTRUCTION OF STATISTICS

Modern health care systems are founded on statistics. The rise of "scientific medicine" since the 1850s is as much a story of statistics as it is of biology or chemistry. Medical practice is shaped by reference to population data—mortality rates, morbidity rates, birth rates, etc.—and by analysis of trial data in the form of the numerical measurement of clinical outcomes. Organizationally, health care management makes wholesale use of numbers in accounting, performance measurement, and the tracking of resource flows. These numbers encode vast amounts of information, reducing this to simple forms that can more easily be manipulated (see Hayek 1945). There is a large research industry devoted to explaining variations in these measures. Qualitative researchers, however, contribute mainly to the study of the encoding process, the decisions that are made in the course of that process about what to count and how to count it, and the implications of these decisions for understanding the eventual outputs. Their findings can help managers, policymakers, and planners evaluate and interpret the quantitative data that are routinely put in front of them, and to make more appropriate decisions about how to act upon these.

Qualitative researchers have long been interested in the organizational production of quantitative data. All statistics rest on definitions about what to count as an example of the phenomenon that they purport to measure. Mortality rates require a prior definition of what counts as a death, for example. Do we mean the cessation of respiration, the absence of a cardiac rhythm, or the lack of detectable electrical activity in the brain?

The study of these processes can tell us a lot about the environment within which health care is delivered. Anleu (2001), for example, examines the history of attempts in Australia to establish a legal definition of the beginning of life. A 1984 statute had regulated research on "embryos." However, scientists were increasingly distinguishing a preembryo period. This lasted from the time at which a sperm penetrated an ovum to the point of syngamy at which the chromosomes unite and a new cell develops. That process lasts about twenty hours and it was not clear whether it was covered by the original legislation. There was a further issue about whether life could be said to exist at this point or not until the emergence of the "primitive streak," the first nerve structure, at about fourteen days. The final legislation, in 1995, produced a definition of the beginning of life, regulating research in these periods but, as Anleu points out, still left areas of ambiguity that are likely to cause future difficulties. The definition simply represents the best available compromise between the prolife, scientific, and therapeutic interests contesting the definition. Law has been used, in the way that it often is, to impose closure "for all practical purposes" on the uncertainties of nature.

Other kinds of quantitative data deal with similar issues. Accountants, for example, need to define when a purchase has been made. Is this when a purchase order is issued, when the goods are delivered, or when the invoice is received and passed? There is no "right answer": the outcome depends on what the information is to be used for. Sometimes it may be important to know what expenditure the organization is committed to, so the significant event is the purchase order. Sometimes, the organization's cash flow is the main concern, so the key information is the point of payment. Law, regulation, and professional conventions are used to structure a flow of activity in particular and more or less arbitrary ways.

Studies of this kind have a strategic relevance to health care personnel. They help to identify issues on which an organization or a profession may need to display particular sensitivity in managing relations with its social, political, or cultural environment. Of greater immediate significance, however, may be studies of how these definitions are used by the people who encode raw information into datasets that display the incidence or prevalence of the various defined events, states, conditions, products, or services and that may be "mined" to identify significant associations between them.

"Official" definitions of what is to be counted are not self-interpreting. They always have to be matched to real cases in real-time situations, often by relatively low-level personnel.[2] This process can lead to unintended but troubling consequences.

The issues were first explored in the course of studies in a Los Angeles psychiatric outpatient clinic, reported by Garfinkel (1967). Data were to be extracted from clinic records to construct successive profiles of a patient cohort, as it passed through intake, psychiatric evaluation, and treatment, in order to identify factors that might affect its attrition. Information would be transferred to a Clinic Career Form that summarized the patient history. However, although some variables were almost always recorded—sex, for example, was noted on 99.5 percent of the files—others were recorded less than one-third of the time. Rather than treating these gaps as evidence of poor performance by the clinic staff, the team came to see them as the consequence of the different uses to which the information was being put. Clinic records were not compiled for the use of researchers but to produce evidence of proper conduct by their authors. They were *contractual*, showing that a job had been performed in a manner that knowledgeable readers of the record would consider appropriate, rather than *actuarial*, a consistent basis of organizational bookkeeping. In fact, the categories that were most fully completed seem to have been those that had to do with billing rather than with therapy, perhaps indicating which matters the organization would pursue if data were found to be missing.

The same team also grappled with the problems of coding the data. The graduate students who had been assigned to this task found that they were constantly having to "make sense" of the record in order to code it. With a limited set of categories and an indefinite set of patients, conditions, and case narratives, the coders had to refashion the events of any particular episode in order to make it into an example of one of the categories that they had available to them. Cicourel (1964) formulated this as the inevitability of measurement by *fiat* (literally, "let it be done"), that measurement always and inevitably involved a prior set of decisions about what would count as an example of what was being measured. Again the outcome was a set of coding sheets that showed they had diligently performed their work rather than a literal summary of the events they had encoded.

These insights have been developed by subsequent studies. Macintyre (1978), for instance, considered the role of records in the intake process for prenatal clinics at a large university hospital. She noted the way in which information-gathering strategies by the intake clerks and nurses were adjusted according to their evaluations of the women being processed. The completion of some sections, especially whether the pregnancy was planned, caused the intake workers some embarrassment. As a result, they would not ask directly for the information or would ask for it apologetically in ways that prompted or assumed particular answers. Nevertheless, once entered, summarized, and analyzed, the results acquired a remarkably hard, factual character:

> Thus, I heard a consultant obstetrician informing a group of nurses in the clinic that 48 per cent of the pregnancies passing through the clinic were unplanned, but that the majority of the women would accommodate to the pregnancy and be quite happy about it. The nurses discussed this information very seriously, even though it was based on their own data collection upon which, in relation to such topics, they do not normally place much reliance, and it appeared to reinforce their belief [used in completing the record entries] that women fundamentally want babies even though they might not have planned their pregnancies. (1978:608)

Like Garfinkel's coders, the nurses interpreted the situation of the women whom they were clerking in order to supply information in the form required by the record. Nevertheless, once this had been recycled into a research finding by the analysis of a senior obstetrician, they accepted the reports as fact and further verification of the commonsense beliefs that they had used initially to deal with the interactional difficulty of asking pregnant women whether they really want to have the baby.[3] Thus reinforced, these beliefs were then used to write future records. More recently, Prior (1985) has looked at the coding of death certificates into mortality statistics in Northern Ireland and the ways in which relatively unskilled clerks made sense of the doctors' descriptions of causes of death and the social data noted on the certificates in order to fit them to the coding rules of the International Classification of Disease. Again the question is raised about the extent to which findings from epidemiological studies of mortality are simply rediscovering patterns created by the coders' stories about these deaths rather than by the population's actual mortality experience.

The recognition that all statistical data are socially and organizationally constructed has often led to a kind of nihilism among qualitative researchers, to the notion that nothing worthwhile can be achieved by quantitative work that rests on such shaky foundations. This has contributed to some of the antagonisms and mutual hostility that we noted earlier in this book. That pushes the problem to an absurd extreme. Clearly important lessons have been learned from quantitative research and its leading practitioners are well aware of the problems outlined above. However, the limits and uncertainties are not always as well understood by users. Lester King, a wise American clinician with an interest in philosophy, has a nice cautionary tale about this. A rather precise young physician joined his lab and asked what they considered the normal hemoglobin level of blood to be:

> When I answered, "twelve to sixteen grams, more or less," he was very puzzled. Most laboratories, he pointed out, called 15 grams normal, or perhaps 14.5. He wanted to know how, if my norm was so broad and vague, he could possibly tell whether a patient suffered from anemia, or how much anemia. I agreed that he had quite a problem on his hands and that it is a very difficult thing to tell. So difficult, in fact, that trying to be too precise is actually misleading, inaccurate, stultifying to thought, and philosophically very unsound.
>
> He wanted to know why I didn't take one hundred or so normal individuals determine their hemoglobin by our method, and use the resulting figure as the normal value for our method. This, I agreed, was a splendid idea. But how were we to pick out the normals? The obvious answer is, just take one or two hundred healthy people, free of disease. ... But that is ex-

actly the difficulty. ... This is traveling in circles, getting us nowhere. (King 1954:194–95)

King's point is that an excess of precision may do more harm than good, in this case leading to either over- or undertreatment. Clinical practice could not be reduced to simple algorithms. In the same way, management is less a matter of rules than of judgment, of knowing what numbers mean rather than being directed by them. The qualitative study of the social construction of quantitative data may be particularly helpful in understanding what the data actually represent, how much weight should be attached to them, and what the consequences of treating them as objective might be. Health care institutions are notoriously difficult to manage by reference to crude performance indicators; work of this kind may help to establish a more sophisticated understanding of the relationship between performance and the instruments by which it is measured. We shall touch on this point again when we look further at the organizational use of records.

REPRESENTATIONS OF ORGANIZATIONS

We have previously referred several times to the pressures on health care organizations and professions from their environment. This is an increasingly important theme in the study of work and organizations, flowing particularly from the work of Meyer and Rowan (1977) and DiMaggio and Powell (1983). Essentially, it is argued that modern organizations and, by implication, professions are required to show that their structures and processes take particular forms if they are to be regarded as "proper" and "legitimate." These pressures increasingly compel them toward isomorphism, looking similar.

Although it does not draw explicitly on this literature, Wiener's (2000) study, introduced in Chapter 2, of the rise of quality assurance in U.S. health care and its impact on two large general hospitals illustrates the argument. She describes the way in which the changing environment of U.S. health care has given rise to increasing pressures for accountability in its delivery. Hospitals have been required to adopt increasingly elaborate internal systems of performance measurement in order to maintain their moral respectability and, hence, their eligibility to receive various types of public or private funding. They are periodically reviewed by accrediting teams, who examine the performance data and interview institutional representatives. Wiener describes the elaborate work that goes into preparation for such visits—drives to complete and update all records, coaching of physicians and nurses who are likely to be interviewed, rewriting of procedural manuals in the accrediting body's preferred format, and so on. The results are only tangentially related to the everyday work of health care providers and the experience of patients. Nevertheless, self-presentation as a rationally managed organization with appropriate datasets, staff buy-in to the mission statement, and the like is crucial to being considered a serious enterprise in contemporary societies (Power 1997).

Such thinking has led to a reappraisal of the traditional skepticism among researchers on organizations and professions about the value of studying the formal aspects of these institutions. The "real" organization was often held to be the underlife revealed by observational studies, where organization members behaved in a variety of ways that would not necessarily be well-regarded by clients but that were critical to its functioning. Dingwall and Strong (1985) reasserted the importance of the ceremonial order of public events and official documents. They were not "mere rhetoric" but symbolic representations of the organization to itself and to outsiders that could reveal what the organization was required to do in order to demonstrate its legitimacy.

These symbolic representations can take various forms. Visual imagery can be important. Dingwall and colleagues showed how the prenatal literature made available to pregnant women in Japan and the United Kingdom transmitted entirely different representations of the "good birth" (Dingwall, Tanaka, & Minamikata 1991). The U.K. National Health Service has recently undergone an expensive rebranding, for example, which, for the first time, has imposed a standard logo on all organizational units that it funds, following earlier moves to impose standardized typography on direction signs and a standardized uniform on nurses. These moves project an aspiration to complete the process of nationalization begun in 1948 and to achieve consistent standards wherever patients encounter the system. Physically, hospital architecture reflects changing theories of medical practice, as much as changing technologies (Prior 1988). Contemporary hospitals do not present themselves to the street as classical temples, in the manner of their nineteenth-century ancestors, but often have more in common with shopping malls.

The study of such imagery is never likely to be a large part of a managerial or policy research agenda but it has some of the same value as the observational studies of institutional low-life. These images may be managed in more or less explicit ways but are always likely to offer important evidence about how policies are being interpreted on the ground. A hospital advertisement, for example, may contain a formal text directed at one audience that is entirely subverted by associated artwork directed at others. Drug advertisements, of course, have long been notorious for this: the mandated information and warnings appear in tiny print alongside a powerful image invoking the benefits.

RECORDS AND MEDICAL WORK

If records are the foundation of both official and organizational statistics, and of quality management systems, they are also intimately linked to the routine performance of frontline health care work. Sometimes, as Dingwall (1977) found in a study of U.K. public health nurses, there is the paradox that not paying much attention to records is a way to demonstrate one's competence as a professional. The "good" nurse knows the personal circumstances of the families with whom she is working so well that she does not need to refer to her records. These are rarely consulted in the course of her work and used only for review by others.

This study predated the large-scale introduction of computerized records in health care systems. In the work introduced in Chapter 3, Greatbatch and colleagues used video recording to explore the way in which computerization affected interaction between doctors and patients. The rational reformers who designed the computer systems took the opportunity to impose structures on the physicians' information collection and recall. Traditional paper records allowed information to be recorded and searched in very free-format ways. In some respects, the more structured approach increased the efficiency of recording and searching. Drug interactions or off-formulary prescribing could be identified, for example, by the checking activities of the software. The records became easier to code for research or quality assurance purposes. However, the nature of the consultation also changed in unexpected ways. Interaction between doctor and patient was subordinated to the demands of data entry, so that physicians gave less attention to patients and patients deferred to the system's requirements. It was harder for the doctor discreetly to review the patient's history by riffling through a folder as the patient talked. Patients seemed to be pressed by the system to present their accounts of signs and symptoms in ways that fitted the record rather than in their own terms, with a possible loss of relevant clinical or social information. The managerial choice of a new recording system had a significant impact on the work of clinicians, the experience of patients, and the nature of the information collected by the practice.

In another context, Rawlings (1989) explores how the sterility of equipment used in surgery is a matter of records as much as of microbiology. She discusses the process of cleaning and sterilizing reusable equipment. The transition from a scalpel being cleaned of, for example, dried blood to being sterile, as a result of autoclaving, was marked by a color change in heat–sensitive sealing tape. No one knew whether the scalpel actually was sterile: sterility was assumed by reference to the indicator tape. This presented a serious problem for an incoming manager who wanted to create a documentary trail that would demonstrate the sterility of equipment in advance of any future challenge. The tape did not do this: all it showed was that the autoclaves were working as well (or as badly) as they usually did. For practical purposes, however, everyone treated it as a reliable indicator because it was all they had, even if it offered no defense against a possible later assertion that the equipment had underperformed. Creating a micro-biologically adequate record would require considerable changes in both technology and working practices.

ORGANIZATIONAL DOCUMENTS

Documents are so central to contemporary health care that they are almost inevitably going to form a major focus for many qualitative studies. In terms of investment of effort and research design, most observational studies will want to look at the interaction between people and texts or images. At the same time, however, it is important to remember that those texts and images are also the *product* of people's work. They are never literal descriptions of reality, even when they appear to relate to such hard and objective phenomena as births and deaths. Laws, regulations, and policies may supply definitions but these always remain to be applied and interpreted often by quite low-level personnel. Compliance with the document-making practices of an organization may be strongly required and heavily sanctioned. This is not, however, going to eliminate the problems of relating documents to action in ways that make sense. It is important to remember the lesson of central planners in the old Soviet Union. If they set output targets for nail factories by weight, they got a small supply of heavy nails. If they set targets by volume, they got a large supply of small nails. Either way, the construction industry did not get the nails it needed to do the job. Qualitative research on the relationship between documented performance and real performance may contribute to avoiding the same problems in contemporary health care.

CONCLUSION

This chapter has reviewed the sources of "given" evidence available to qualitative researchers, whether by means of direct observation, audio and video recording, or in the form of statistics, images, and documents. While these represent the preferred sources of data, it must also be acknowledged that they are not always achievable. Some events happen in ways that make them difficult to capture by means of these research technologies. Sometimes, quicker and cheaper information is required, even if it is less accurate or of lesser evidential value. The next chapter will look at the main solution to this problem in the form of the qualitative interview.

NOTES

1. The ethics of qualitative research are discussed in Chapter 8. Although this might imply that Millman did not get informed consent from patients, remember that they are incidental to her study. This focuses on the doctors and other staff who had consented to their work being observed. A contemporary investigator might put more stress on actually being introduced to patients as a researcher but it must be stressed that participant observers have limited control over the behavior of the people they are studying. Indeed, the whole point of observation is to minimize disruption and if staff do not normally consider it necessary to introduce students or junior colleagues working with them, then this may be data for the study rather than something that a fieldworker can or should expect to affect.

2. Even if the process is automated, as with the traces generated by equipment in intensive care or by in the printouts from testing machines, the recording represents the outcome of past human decisions, creating an "inscription device" whose uniformity belies the original basis of judgment on which it was designed (Latour & Woolgar 1979).

3. This is an everyday version of the problems discussed in Chapter 5 about the status of interview data.

5

Interviews in Qualitative Research

There is a growing interest in qualitative interviews as an alternative to the standardized interviews that are well-established as a research technique. Indeed, judging by the contents of health studies journals, qualitative interviews seem, for many, to be synonymous with qualitative research. They are used to elicit consumer evaluations of health care, to uncover patient and professional models of health and illness, and to explore patients' experiences of illness. They can also be found in studies of the rationales underpinning patient concordance and nonconcordance with prescribed treatment and of the relationships between different health occupations, on the one hand, and between professionals and patients on the other. This chapter begins with a description of what qualitative interviews are. We consider when interview methods might be used instead of observation, which, as we explained in the previous chapter, would generally be considered the "gold standard" for qualitative research. We then explain why qualitative interviews are sometimes more useful than quantitative ones. Finally, we discuss some of the limitations of qualitative interview data.

WHAT ARE QUALITATIVE INTERVIEWS?

The term "qualitative interview" covers a broad range of activities. Traditionally, qualitative interviews have been encounters between a single interviewer and a single informant.[1] However, group interviews or focus groups have become increasingly popular (see, for example, Morgan 1992; Halloran & Grimes 1995). These methods are particularly useful when the object of the research is to tease out group norms and assumptions that may often not be talked about explicitly in everyday practice (Bloor, Frankland, Thomas, & Robson 2001).

Qualitative methods texts propose various typologies of qualitative interview. For example, Denzin distinguished between "non-schedule" standardized interviews in which "the interviewer works with a list of the information required from each respondent" (1970:125) but the particular phrasing and ordering of questions is adapted to suit individual informants, and "non-standardized" interviews in which no specific set of questions is employed and questions are not asked in any particular order. More recently, Grbich (1999) distinguished between "informal," "guided," and "structured open-ended" interviews. Informal interviews are defined as casual conversations that arise spontaneously, generally in the context of an observational study. Guided interviews involve a set of broad-ranging questions, derived from previous studies or the researcher's experience, which the interviewer is free to order, phrase, and present at his or her own discretion. In structured, open-ended interviews, the same questions are asked in the same sequence but informants are encouraged to answer these questions in their own terms and, where appropriate, to expand on their initial responses.

The proliferation of typologies reflects their limited usefulness. It is more helpful to think of qualitative interviews as ranged along a continuum in terms of the degree of control the researcher seeks to exert over the content and structure of the encounter. At one extreme, the researcher may simply introduce a broad topic and invite the informant to contribute without overtly seeking to constrain or direct the talk. At the other, the researcher comes to the interview with a clear set of issues to be examined in the interview and, in some cases, a list of questions to introduce each issue. The decision about where to locate the interviews in any particular study along this continuum should be guided by the research questions being asked and the current state of knowledge in the field in question. If a local issue is being explored in the context of a significant body of existing knowledge, then a more structured approach is appropriate, as the researcher tries to identify similarities and differences. On the other hand, if there is little previous literature—on patient responses to physical therapy, for example—a more open approach is indicated.

In both group and individual contexts, interviewers use a variety of stimuli to elicit talk about the topic they are investigating. Asking questions remains the most usual approach, but other techniques are emerging. For example, interviewers may ask their informants to respond to vignettes. These are stories about individuals and situations. Typically informants are asked to describe how they themselves would respond to the same situation or, in some cases, to say how they think a third party would respond. Hughes (1998) describes the use of this technique in a study of drug injectors who had spent some time in prison. The aim of the study was to explore experiences of prison and HIV risk and safer behavior. A lengthy (thousand-word) vignette was presented to informants in a storybook format. This vignette followed the lives and experiences of two main characters as they moved in and out of the prison system. The reading of the story was punctuated by questions, asking the informants to consider what might happen next and whether they themselves had ever found themselves in a similar situation. Vignettes offer the opportunity for informants to discuss issues in a nonpersonal and possibly less threatening context. Data derived from vignettes cannot, of course, be treated as indications of what informants would *actually* do if faced with the same situation in real life. They can, however, help to elicit the starting assumptions or frameworks with which people address the issue under consideration.

For many purposes, we can also think of "elicited documents" like health diaries, activity reports and visualizations as forms of interview. Here, we are thinking of documents that research participants are asked to produce in the knowledge that they will be read by the researcher, although not by other organization members. In effect, they display their authors' responses to the starting questions or briefing given by the researcher on a longer term basis than a specific interview. Although we shall not discuss these forms of data more specifically in this chapter, most of what is said about interview data and its status also applies to them.

WHEN ARE INTERVIEWS THE METHOD OF CHOICE?

There are some circumstances where interviews have significant advantages over observation (Kleinman, Stenross, & McMahon 1994). Some questions of interest to research consumers are simply not amenable to observational research. Relevant activity does not always take place in neatly definable geographical locations such as a hospital ward, clinic, or doctor's office. Mathieson and Stam (1995), for example, analyzed the narrative concepts produced in the course of open-ended interviews with cancer patients. While patients might, from time to time, produce such narratives spontaneously during everyday interactions, there is no predictable time or place when they routinely do so. The researcher would need to observe the patient for an inordinately long period of time to secure a relatively small amount of data. Elicitation in an interview is the most practical option.

Some things only happen in places that are private rather than public or semipublic, so that researchers are unlikely to gain the extended access that is necessary for observational studies. There is, for example, a growing appreciation that much health work is carried out by unwaged carers in the privacy of their own homes. This includes not only nursing care of sick, elderly, and disabled family members, but also routine monitoring of the health status of children and the provision of food and other forms of care. While observational studies of such settings may, occasionally, be possible (see, for example, Douglas & Nicod, 1974), few families will tolerate this kind of sustained intrusion into their everyday lives. In such cases, interviews are, again, likely to be the most efficient way of collecting relevant data (see, for example, Gantley, Davies, & Murcott 1993; Murphy 1999, 2000; Lauritzen 1997). Similarly, there is a long, if not large-scale, tradition of life-history studies in social science, where a single individual, or group of individuals, recounts the story of their life, which may then be used as a case study to examine some more general issue. Again one needs to consider the impracticality of lifelong observation. This has had relatively little application in health studies but influential examples in other areas of social research would include Shaw (1966), Klockars (1974), and Lewis (1961).

Researchers may be excluded from observation in other settings by lack of the relevant membership qualifications, including professional certification, age, gender, or ethnicity. The activities in which they have a legitimate interest may also be so private or stigmatized that they are impossible to observe. For example, it is difficult to imagine how Rhodes and Cusick (2000) could have obtained data on the negotiation of safety in sexual relationships between HIV positive drug users and their partners other than through interviews.

In some cases, then, interviewing may be the only practical technique for investigating a particular topic. However, interviews also have other uses, particularly when used alongside observational methods. As we noted in the previous chapter, most observational studies incorporate interviews into their research design. Often these will be informal discussions between the observer and participants that arise in the course of the observation. At other times, they will be more formal encounters that are negotiated in advance with interviewees. Both formal and informal interviews make an important contribution to observational studies. They can offer an opportunity to compare researchers' interpretations of what they have seen and heard with those of the participants or of other members of the groups involved (Denscombe 1983). They can draw the observer's attention to aspects of the setting that might otherwise be overlooked. In some cases, interviews are also used to collect comparative or supplementary data on a greater number of settings or groups than would be feasible using observational methods alone (see, for example, Guillemin & Holmstrom 1986).

Interviews are also sometimes chosen for entirely pragmatic reasons. It is generally easier to negotiate access for them than for extended periods of observation, especially with unsophisticated institutional review boards.[2] They can be conveniently scheduled to meet the time constraints of both interviewer and informant, a useful consideration, especially where researchers are attempting to combine a study with teaching or clinical practice. Interview studies tend to be cheaper and quicker to complete. However, as so often in research, these benefits are gained at a price. Often interviews are invitations to informants to serve as proxy observers, describing events or their own internal experiences and states of mind. The descriptions of events are secondhand and produced by an untrained observer whose selection and organization of the report introduces unknown influences before the researcher begins analysis. This is the "double transformation" discussed in Chapter 4. Similarly, descriptions of the informant's internal experiences reconstruct these for the purposes of the interview. Interview data inject the informant's interpretations and inferences before the researcher ever gets to work. Such a lengthening of the chain of interpretation and inference does not necessarily mean that interview data are irredeemably flawed but it does mean that we need to be particularly careful in what we do with them. We shall come back to this point later.

WHY NOT STICK TO STANDARDIZED INTERVIEWS?

The growing enthusiasm for qualitative interviewing in health studies partly arises from disillusionment with the results of using the highly standardized interview techniques typical of survey research. These techniques aim to elicit objective facts from respondents (whether these are reports of events, of opinions, or of attitudes), while ensuring that these are not contaminated by the interview procedures. Typically, the interviewer is required to ask exactly the same questions, in exactly the same way, of all respondents. Question wording and question order are both decided in advance. Interviewers are warned to stick strictly to the script and to avoid any variation in self-presentation or behavior that might bias interviewees' responses. The underlying logic is that, if the conduct of the interview is identical for all respondents, then we can be confident that any differences between them that are uncovered in the analysis are *real* differences rather than artifacts of the interview. From this perspective, interviews are a means of gathering facts about reality, whether that reality exists externally in the world or internally in the respondent's mind.

The difficulty is that standardized interviewer behavior and self-presentation does not guarantee standardization of response. Survey interviewers are faced with two fundamentally incompatible imperatives (Cicourel 1964). On the one hand, they are supposed to administer the questionnaire in an identical way to all respondents. On the other, they are urged to build rapport in order to create an atmosphere in which respondents will feel able to offer frank responses to the questions asked. In effect, the researcher is required to adapt to each respondent but, at the same time, is constrained to act in an identical fashion with each one. There is, at the very least, considerable tension between these two goals. The former implies that the ideal interviewer behaves like an automaton. The second calls for the exercise of the flexible social skills routinely displayed in everyday social interactions where each party adapts to the mood, appearance, and so on of the other. Cicourel sums up the problem:

> If the interviewer were like a robot with built-in speaking and tape recording equipment, this would insure standardization and insure the researcher that standardized stimuli are being presented to the subject, but it would not allow any flexibility in the presentation of self. (ibid.:90–91)

Interviews are social situations to which *both* participants bring their own expectations, experiences, and notions of proper behavior. The interaction will be colored by the participants' perceptions of "their attractiveness or unattractiveness to one another, their bodily presence, the social, physical and role difference" (ibid.:80).

However much researchers may seek to control the interviewer's input, they cannot standardize the interaction between that and the framing that the respondent brings to the encounter.[3] In answering questions, respondents are always involved in a process of interpretation. Simply administering an identically worded question to all respondents does not guarantee that they will all hear and interpret it in an identical fashion. Advocates of a less standardized approach argue for a shift away from standardizing questions to seeking "equivalence of meaning" (Richardson, Dohrenwend, & Klein 1966). Interviewers should be encouraged to tailor questions to the vocabulary and understandings of individual respondents, rather than to seek to impose a uniform set of stimuli regardless of variations in the way that they are understood.

In practice, whether standardized questions cause serious problems depends upon the extent to which there is a reasonably standard understanding of their topics. If we want to know something about the social demography of a hospital's catchment population, for example, most people in the United States and other developed countries will understand and answer questions about their age and date of birth in a uniform fashion. However, these are not socially relevant data for people in many other societies and this causes difficulties when migrants are asked the same questions. A study of Pakistani women using obstetric services in an English city, for example, found a high prevalence of 1 January birth dates being recorded by the intake staff using a formal questionnaire (Bowler 1995). Birthdays were not important events for this particular group, but the women had discovered that they needed to supply an answer to this question when dealing with English officialdom.[4]

If we go back to the example of the hypothetical study of clinic waiting time and patient satisfaction, introduced in Chapter 2, then we can see that waiting time may not be difficult to record, given the near-universal metric of "clock time." However, the equivalence of the meaning of ratings on a satisfaction scale cannot be so easily assumed. At a minimum, this is likely to be affected by prior notions of what counts as a "reasonable" wait, by what happens during the waiting period, and by the outcome of the visit. Notions of a "reasonable wait" may be colored by other experiences or the place of the clinic visit in the patient's other activities for the day. Someone who is retired or not employed may be much more tolerant of waiting than those who are losing income, either because they are self-employed or because they are not in a salaried job. There are ways of dealing with these problems within the standardized interview approach but the more concerned we are with patients' own perceptions of their experiences, the more appropriate qualitative work becomes. Having said this, a recurrent theme in the argument of Chapters 3 and 4 has been the difficulty of simply assuming that qualitative interviews give us access to those perceptions.

THE QUALITATIVE ALTERNATIVE

The advantages often claimed for qualitative approaches to interviewing invert the critique of standardized interviews. Qualitative interviews are seen as an opportunity to explore how informants themselves define the experiences and practices that are the object of the research. Unlike standardized interviews, they are said not to impose a "pre-defined 'grid' of categories assumed to represent the range of possible alternative responses appropriate to the area of research" (Voysey 1975:66).

Mathieson and Stam (1995) contrast their approach to understanding the experiences of people living with cancer with more traditional standardized research in psychosocial oncology. They suggest that such research relies on measures of psychosocial outcomes derived from the medical model "in an attempt to *classify* patients according to their emotional reactions to cancer" (ibid.:285, emphasis in original). Other frequently used measures of "adaptation" or "adjustment" are derived from the cognitive adaptation model. In either case, they argue, the models are highly individualistic, assuming that people react to cancer in isolation from previous social experiences and current networks. As such, the models may have little relevance to the "lived experience of a chronic, life-threatening disease" (ibid.:286). In Voysey's terms, such approaches risk imposing an inappropriate grid upon patients' experiences (Voysey 1975).

The approach adopted by Mathieson and Stam was somewhat different.

They interviewed a total of thirty-seven people with various cancers, using a range of open-ended questions. The questions were informed by the findings of two previous studies, one concerned primarily with identity issues and the other focusing upon the concerns of cancer patients. On average, the interviews lasted two hours. They were audio-recorded and most were transcribed. In analyzing the transcripts, the authors identified the ways in which people talked about themselves at various stages of their cancer, focusing upon the identity problems that were precipitated by the condition. In the early stages of the disease, informants referred to discrepancies between their former healthy lives and their lives as "people with cancer." These discrepancies arose *both* from physical changes *and* from changes in social relationships and disruptions to daily routines resulting from medical interventions. Faced with this disruption of their identity, cancer patients had to reevaluate themselves within the constraints of both the stigma associated with the condition and the dominance of the institutional demands of medicine. In the course of the interviews, patients engaged in what Mathieson and Stam call "biographical work" as they talked about their illness, retrospectively redefining their past as well as projecting their future.

Mathieson and Stam's study is an attempt to "view the culture of illness from the lives of the ill rather than from the perspective of the researcher or the medical system" (1995:302). For McCracken, such penetration of the minds of informants is the key characteristic of qualitative interviews:

> The method can take us into the mental world of the individual, to glimpse the categories and logic by which he or she sees the world. It can also take us into the life world of the individual, to see the content and pattern of daily experience. The long interview gives us the opportunity to step into the mind of another person, to see and experience the world as they do themselves. (1988:9)

To use the language we introduced in Chapter 2, interviews are a means of *verstehen* or of taking the role of the other.

Advocates of qualitative interviews often point to the policy relevance of the insights that can be gained if we avoid imposing our own structures and assumptions upon informants' views of the world (Britten 1995). Quantitative interviews may run a serious risk of misleading policy and practice by failing to uncover the range and depth of people's feelings and opinions (Pill 1995). Uncovering informants' beliefs, understandings, and cultures can be an important way to test the assumptions of researchers, practitioners, and policymakers. However, as we have already observed at several points, it is not straightforward to treat data from qualitative interviews as giving unproblematic access to informants' "authentic" meanings and experiences. Mathieson and Stam recognize this problem:

> These conversations are colored by the position of patient versus researcher, narrator and listener, question and answer, yet the narrative is a combination of the intended and unintended consequences of the interaction. (1995:283)

Unfortunately, having acknowledged the point, Mathieson and Stam then appear to proceed with their analysis *as if* the narratives coproduced in this way do indeed represent *the* meaning of events and experiences to their informants. Later in this chapter we look more deeply at the problems of analyzing interview data.

A second advantage that is often proposed for qualitative interviews relates to the degree of flexibility that they offer. As we saw in Chapter 3, such flexibility is characteristic of qualitative research design more generally. This makes qualitative interviews particularly useful in situations where there is little prior knowledge about the topic under investigation. In standardized interviews, the researcher is required to know in advance what the interesting and relevant dimensions of the topic are and to translate these into clearly specified questions, the "pre-defined grid" referred to earlier. By contrast, in qualitative studies, the researcher is free to follow up interesting leads and to open up new dimensions as they arise during the data collection. This is greatly facilitated where the analysis of the interview data is carried out alongside the ongoing data collection.

The qualitative research literature offers numerous examples to illustrate the benefits of such flexibility in research design. One is Svensson's (1996) study of the interplay between doctors and nurses in Swedish hospitals. As Svensson acknowledges, this interview study was originally designed to investigate "the empirical validity and possibilities for further development of the doctor-nurse game" (ibid.:382). This is a reference to an influential earlier paper by a U.S. physician, Leonard Stein (1967; see also Stein et al. 1990), based on his own clinical experiences: His data are essentially observational, even if they are anecdotal rather than systematic. He noted how interactions between doctors and nurses were permeated by doctors' dominant status and need for omnipotence. Nurses were only able to exert influence indirectly through a "doctor-nurse game" that enabled them to inform and advise doctors without directly challenging their status. The game was a potential source of communication failures, with implications for patient safety or well-being, if either party was not sufficiently skillful in dealing with its indirectness. As Svensson's data collection proceeded, it became clear that this framework did not fit well with the data that were emerging from the interviews. These suggested that the interaction between doctors and nurses was very different to that reported by Stein. The nurses interviewed by Svensson stated that they had little difficulty conveying their ideas and opinions to doctors, and that these were listened to and taken into account. As these findings emerged, Svensson adjusted the focus of his study to take account of them, exploring the ways in which nurses actively engaged in negotiations with the doctors. As we show later, Svensson's interpretation of his data is open to question, but the change of direction is typical of the inherent flexibility of qualitative research.

A further argument put forward in support of qualitative interviews is that they are more likely to generate a truthful account from informants (Denzin 1970). This claim rests upon two assumptions. The first is that, compared to standardized interviews, qualitative interviews offer a context in which the interviewer is more likely to be able to establish a positive and comfortable relationship with the informant. The more relaxed interactions that can be established in qualitative interviews probably do encourage the development of greater rapport and intimacy between informant and interviewer. However, it is not clear that this will necessarily lead to greater openness and truthfulness. Certainly one would expect the two types of interview to be different, just as is the case with more or less intimate conversations in everyday life. A distinction between public and private accounts (Cornwell 1984) is sometimes used to signal the relationship between the context of the interview and the data obtained. There is, though, no particular reason to assume that qualitative interviews generate "private accounts." When carrying out qualitative interviews with child protective services directors, for example, Dingwall found that they tended to treat him as if he were a journalist from the local news media. Whatever lower level managers might say about the "real life" of the agencies, the directors had well-rehearsed public accounts of how well everything worked. This is not, of course, to suggest that those interviews were useless as data: merely that we need to understand exactly what sort of data they are. However, as we show later, this takes us a long way from claiming that the accounts produced in the course of qualitative interviews are more accurate, particularly when one is dealing with sensitive or stigmatized topics. Indeed, one might argue that, having established a relationship with the interviewer, the informant would have even more reason to be concerned about the impression that he or she is making than in the rather more anonymous and impersonal context of a standardized interview.

The important point here is that *all* interview talk, like all other naturally occurring talk, is *always* socially and contextually constrained. What we say and how we say it is never divorced from the context in which we say it. All interactions, whether for the purposes of research or not, involve what Dingwall (1997) has described as a "dance of expectations." The basic features of this dance are as follows:

I produce my actions in the expectation that you will understand them in a particular way. Your understanding reflects your expectations of what would be a proper action for me in these particular circumstances which, in turn, becomes the basis of your response which, itself, reflects your expectations of how I will respond. And so on. At any point, there may be a disjuncture between actions, responses and expectations which requires that the parties engage in some sort of repair work. (ibid.:56)

Interviews are inevitably occasions for "impression management" (Goffman 1959), where all parties—informants *and* interviewers alike—strive to present themselves as competent, sane, and moral persons to those with whom they are interacting. What are the consequences of this?

WHAT KIND OF INFORMATION CAN
WE GET FROM INTERVIEW DATA?

This acknowledgment of the interactional dynamics of interviews has important implications for the ways in which researchers can properly use the data generated. Some of these implications are still being worked out and you should not expect every interview study fully to reflect them, especially if it was carried out some years ago. Nevertheless, you should aim to ask whether the issues discussed in this section affect the analysis and conclusions that are reported. If they had been acknowledged, would the report look different? Interview data are used for a range of purposes and we shall consider the relationship between these data and the circumstances under which they are produced for each purpose.

Reporting on External Reality

This may be the most obvious use of interview data. The researcher asks the informant to provide information about some event, usually one that the researcher did not personally observe. The informant plays the role of proxy observer, supplying information about what was done or said on that occasion, whether by the informant or by others. What status should we give to the informant's report?

If we adopt the subtle realist position proposed in Chapter 1, there is no problem in treating such reports as *potentially* accurate descriptions of the occurrences that they report. Clearly these reports are a product of an interaction between what actually happened and the frameworks available to the informant for "making sense" of it and talking about it to an interviewer. Different informants may, of course, use different frameworks to observe and report on the same event. This means that it is possible to have several different versions of that event, each of which is true for the observer who produced it. However, they are different versions *of the same event*, which means that they can legitimately be examined *both* as evidence of that event *and* as evidence of the way in which different observers have come to understand and talk about it.

While we can never know with absolute certainty that an informant's report is true, we can evaluate it rigorously. This allows us to make an informed judgment about its trustworthiness. Such evaluation can be done in a number of ways. The first and most obvious approach is to form a judgment about whether or not the informant could be expected to have access to the information that he or she is reporting. It is surprising how often this apparently simple imperative is overlooked. For example, in a paper concerned with patient responses to benzodiazepine medication, Diana North and her colleagues state that "general practitioners gave these participants a high degree of autonomy to self-medicate within guidelines" (North, Davis, & Powell 1995:641). This conclusion was supported by the following extract from their patient interview data.

> He's got confidence in me to make the right decisions and not sort of ... I'm sure he doesn't think I'm relying totally on drugs ... and I'm sure if he did he wouldn't ever allow me that freedom to make that ... I'm sure that he would have directed me more than he has done. (ibid.:642)

The accuracy of the patient's report depends crucially upon the transparency of the doctor's mental processes and motivations, but the authors do not appear to question this patient's assertion that she has access to these.

A second means of evaluating informants' reports depends upon the possibility of cross-checking data on the same event from different informants. As we have already observed, we would not expect identical reports from different observers. It is entirely possible to have multiple, noncompeting, valid descriptions of the same phenomenon (Hammersley & Atkinson 1995). However, what is not possible is to have multiple *contradictory* descriptions that are nonetheless all valid. This suggests that research consumers need to be particularly careful in drawing conclusions from studies that rely exclusively on reports from one party to an event or interaction. Once again, it is surprising how often this problem is overlooked. In Svensson's (1996) study of the interplay between doctors and nurses, which was introduced above, the author concluded that the social order on medical and surgical wards was the result of continuous negotiation between doctors and nurses. He reported that nurses had "increased their influence over decisions which affect the patient, and they can influence the norms for interaction and work performance to a greater extent than previously. On the wards covered by this study, the voice of nursing clearly makes itself heard in more areas and with greater strength than it did before" (ibid.:306). This sweeping conclusion is based entirely upon data derived from interviews with nurses. There is no attempt to discover whether the other party to these interactions (the doctors) reported the same radical shift in doctor-nurse relationships.

Svensson himself recognizes the relatively fragile foundation for his findings when he comments,

> It is important to point out that the present analysis ... is based on interview data. ... Our interviews with nurses have given us insights into their reflections on their relationships with doctors. At the same time, the reliability of subjective accounts of this sort can always be questioned. To find out about how negotiations are conducted, how people actually behave towards each other in different types of situations one should not rely solely upon actor's own accounts. (ibid.:396)

The force of Svensson's caveat becomes clearer if we compare the findings from his study with those of Allen (1997). Like Svensson, Allen was interested in the division of labor between doctors and nurses and, in particular, in negotiation of interoccupational boundaries. Allen used a range of methods in her study. She collected data through participant observation on the wards of a nine-hundred-bed general hospital, nursing and management meetings, and in-service study days. In addition to her observations, she also carried out fifty-seven tape-recorded interviews and a number of spontaneous extended conversations with staff, as well as analyzing organizational documents.

It is clear, from both the interview and the observational data, that interoccupational boundaries were a salient issue for both doctors and nurses. Hospital managers encouraged nurses to extend their skills in numerous areas including administration of intravenous antibiotics, venepuncture, ECGs, male catheterization, and intravenous cannulation. Both doctors and nurses appeared to be somewhat equivocal about the devolution of medical tasks to nurses and there were divergent perspectives concerning interoccupational boundaries. In her formal and informal interviews, Allen found some support for Svensson's conclusion that nurses were more actively negotiating and contesting their boundaries with doctors. She reports: "In my conversations and interviews with staff many recounted instances of contested boundaries" (ibid.:505).

The nurses stressed their control over attempts by doctors to delegate medical tasks to them. They insisted that their priority was to carry out traditional nursing care. If they were busy with nursing tasks and doctors wanted to devolve a medical task to them they would expect to negotiate the allocation of work.

Her observations, however, showed little evidence of such negotiation:

Nevertheless, my field observations revealed that on the wards, nursing, medical and support staff carried out their work activities with minimal inter-occupational negotiation and little explicit conflict. (ibid.)

Contrary to the nurses' accounts of their working practices, Allen found that nurses undertook doctor-devolved work irrespective of the other work pressures that they were experiencing. Moreover, they routinely violated organizational policies by undertaking a whole range of activities such as ordering additional intravenous fluids, requesting standard blood tests, initiating referrals, giving saline flushes after the administration of antibiotics, and administering drugs without a prescription, when doctors were unavailable on the wards.

How are we to understand this discrepancy between nurses' accounts of their work, with their emphasis on nurse control of the boundary between medical and nursing work, and Allen's firsthand observations that suggested that nurses rarely exercised such control or engaged in face-to-face negotiations with doctors? Allen suggests that it may be more appropriate to treat nurses' interview accounts as "displays of perspectives or moral forms" (ibid.:514) rather than literal representations of reality. From this position, the nurses' talk can be seen as resisting "the charge that they were being 'dumped on' by the medical profession wishing to discard their 'dirty work'" (ibid.:505). The nurses are *making a claim* about themselves and their work *as well as describing* their relationship with medical staff. The description is structured by the claim rather than being a literal rendering of the events to which it refers.

All this points to the importance of treating interview talk as social action. In evaluating any interview report, a key question to ask is, "What is the informant *doing* with their interview talk?" (Silverman 1993). Qualitative interviews are sometimes described as "conversations with a purpose" but the informant's purpose may not necessarily be identical to that of the researcher. Indeed, one might well expect that informants would be juggling a number of different purposes in the interview and that the data obtained would be the outcome of their interplay. The accurate representation of reality is only one of the goals toward which informants may be expected to orient themselves during an interview. Alternative purposes might include both micropolitical projects and favorable self-presentation.

We cannot assume that informants are naive about the potential micropolitical impact of research findings. Indeed, one motivation for agreeing to take part in an interview study may be a desire to ensure that their perspective, or that of their group, is adequately and favorably represented. Patients are often eager to provide a "patient's-eye-view" of medical services, or of everyday life with a particular disease, in the hope of reforming services or making health professionals and policymakers more sensitive to their needs. Under such conditions, interview data will be the product of the tension between offering the interviewer an accurate report of reality and a concern to present that reality in a way that contributes to the micropolitical project.

This is further complicated by self-presentation, which is a pervasive feature of all social interactions, whether research interviews or naturally occurring conversations. Participants in social interaction are concerned with how they appear to others. When we respond to requests for reports on our own behavior, or that of others, we routinely consider the possible inferences that might be drawn from those reports about the behavior they describe. We are aware that much of our behavior is, at least potentially, open to question, when viewed from particular perspectives. Thus, in the context of nursing ideologies that stress the autonomy and independence of nurses, clearing up a mess left by a doctor could be seen as evidence of servility or a lack of proper self-respect. The reports offered by such nurses in interview situations are likely to be edited to defend against such inferences.

The significance of this perspective on interview reports as social action is underscored by a number of studies that have reported the occurrence of so-called atrocity stories in health care settings. The term "atrocity story" was coined by Stimson and Webb (1975) in their classic study of doctor-patient consultations in British general practice. Like Allen (1997), they combined observations of actual consultations with group and individual interviews, although, for practical reasons, they were unable to interview the particular patients whom they had observed interacting with doctors in consultations. Nevertheless, Stimson and Webb were struck by the discrepancies between the ways that patients described their interactions with doctors in interviews and the researchers' own observations of such encounters. In the consultations they observed, patients were almost uniformly passive and apparently compliant:

> Patients rarely give open expression to feelings of disagreement or dissatisfaction to the doctor's face but may mask them behind muttered or mumbled comments which are barely audible. (1975:53)

In the course of the interviews, however, much of the patients' talk involved vivid descriptions of their encounters with doctors. Although some of these stories involved praising individual doctors, most were critical, which was why the researchers came to call them "atrocity stories." Patients typically portrayed themselves as playing a very active part in the encounter. This is one example:

My daughter turned round and said: "Look doctor, if you don't get him out of here right away I will go right over your head." Her boss told her to say that. He was gone. "You will have an ambulance right away." Well, within ten minutes the ambulance was here. (ibid.:97)

Atrocity stories had a number of recurrent features. Very often the patient was presented as having dominated the exchange. Where the story involved a dispute between doctor and patient, it often concluded with a report of how the patient's view was vindicated by later events. Doctors were frequently presented as callous, inhumane, or incompetent. They might be described in derogatory language that made them appear foolish or laughable.

Once again, we see the discrepancy between observations and reports, the consultations witnessed by Stimson and Webb and the accounts given by patients in research interviews. We suggested that a key question to ask in relation to interview data concerns what the informants might be *doing* with their talk. Stimson and Webb (1975) offered one possible interpretation. They suggested that the telling of atrocity stories was one way in which patients could redress the inequalities that are inherent in a relationship where the doctor dispenses services and the patient requires some action to be taken on his or her behalf. The stories told by both Svensson's nurses and Stimson and Webb's patients cast them as people who were "proper" and "competent" performers of a particular social role: nurses who were not the organizational inferiors of physicians and patients who were self-directed consumers of medicine rather than passive and deferential dependents on professional authority.

Such "storytelling" appears to be very common when people are interviewed about their encounters with health professionals. In some cases (see, for example, Baruch 1981), the researcher is careful to consider the work that such stories are being made to do by the informant. In others, the researcher appears to treat such stories as offering a literal description of some encounter between health professional and patient. Earlier in this chapter, we discussed Mathieson and Stam's (1995) interview study, where they explored patients' "identity work" in the narratives they produced during the interviews. Among the data reproduced are a number of excerpts that seem to be atrocity stories. For example, one patient reported:

So I got the second round (of chemotherapy), and I was half way through that when I was really getting beaten into the ground, and I said, "Look, I was told half a year ago that this was not the route to go with cervical cancer. Now why are you doing this?" and so that's when he admitted, "We don't know how to treat you," and ... I told him, "Please don't ever do that to me again. I don't mind not knowing something. ... " So he spent three-quarters of an

hour with me, and you know what he says? "There should be more conversations like this." I said, "*You* have to instigate this. We are dealing with a very
dramatic situation here, and *you're* telling *me* there should be more conversations like this?" (ibid.:298)

This story shows many of the features characteristic of atrocity stories.
The doctor is at fault. The patient takes control. She does not demand the
impossible. She shows understanding of the doctor's inability to offer informed advice about the best course of action. In spite of his shortcomings,
she responds with courtesy but she does not fail to point out his faults. Her
stance is vindicated by the doctor's acknowledgment of his failings and his
aspiration to do better in the future. However, in spite of their declared
commitment to interpreting interview data as "joint action" (ibid.:284),
Mathieson and Stam treat this as a direct report on an interaction with her
doctor. In their article, they introduce this data extract as follows:

> Several seasoned patients in our study also provided striking examples of
> attempts to negotiate as equal partners within medical discourse. A woman
> with Stage IV cervical cancer described this as a "transition into shared space."
> Her dialogue with her oncologist in the excerpt below suggests that the
> emergence of patient voice reflects the cumulative effect of living with an
> illness. (ibid.:298)

Having presented the report, they offer the following comment, implicitly assuming the factual status of the story:

> To deny a patient her voice, or to promote a system which does not permit
> the development of voice, threatens identity because it conveys to the indi-
> vidual that there is no need to personally evaluate the illness experience.
> (ibid.:298–99)

If a paper like this is read uncritically, it can easily be taken to be evidence of continuing failures of communication between physicians and
patients. However, if we are right and patients are, in some sense, constrained to report their interaction with physicians in ways that stress
physician failures, then real improvements in communication will go unnoticed, unrecorded, and unacknowledged. It is quite possible for a
transformation in medical practice to be obscured by an interactional expectation that patients will present themselves as active and sophisticated
consumers.

In the next section, we turn to a second use of interview data. Here we
move from considering interview reports as representations of external
reality to considering them as representations of the internal reality of the
person being interviewed.

Experiences, Meaning, and Motivations

One of the most frequent claims for qualitative interviews is that they allow researchers to explore the ways in which informants themselves define the experiences and practices that are the focus of the research (Paget 1983; Merriam 1988; Crabtree & Miller 1991; de Vries, Weijts, Dijkstra, & Kok 1992; Britten 1995). In contrast to quantitative interviews they open up the possibility of challenging the researcher's preconceptions about what is important or significant. They are a means of discovering "the insider's perspective" (Jensen 1989), "how research participants understand their world" (Secker, Wimbush, Watson, & Milburn 1995), or the informant's "frame of reference" (Oiler Boyd 1993b; Britten 1995). Patton identified this as one of the key advantages of interviews when compared with observational methods:

> We cannot observe feelings, thoughts and intentions. ... We cannot observe how people have organized the world and the meanings they attach to what goes on in the world—we have to ask people questions about those things. The purpose of interviewing, then, is to allow us to enter into the other person's perspective. (1980:196)

All these authors see the skillful use of qualitative interviews as a way of uncovering the meanings, beliefs, understandings, and cultures of informants.

The attraction to health researchers of uncovering participant understandings and perspectives is obvious. It is widely assumed that trouble in medical settings arises when there is a breakdown in understanding of the perspectives of others. For example, nurses are thought not to understand what it is like to be a doctor and vice versa. Both have difficulty in putting themselves in the shoes of patients or managers. Qualitative interviews are seen as a way of uncovering the perspectives of these different groups and, as a result, of exposing each group to the thinking of the others.

We have no problem with the idea that interviews can challenge taken-for-granted assumptions or introduce aspects of a situation that were previously opaque. This potential is illustrated, for example, by Morgan and Watkins's (1988) study of the beliefs and responses to hypertensive medication in different cultural groups. The authors were concerned about improving understanding of patient responses to hypertension and to advice about its management. They used qualitative interviews to elicit beliefs and concerns about hypertension that were current among white and African-Caribbean people who had been diagnosed with this condition for at least one year. These interviews uncovered a practice of "leaving off" medication that was current among their African-Caribbean informants. This practice involved not taking medication for periods of time in order to avoid dependency, mixing alcohol and prescribed drugs, or taking medication when they had no symptoms.

However, the idea that interviews can uncover otherwise inaccessible rationales and cultural assumptions current in subgroups of the community is too often confused with the claim that they are a means to discover why people behave as they do. This claim incorporates at least two questionable assumptions.

First, there is the assumption that, inside informants' heads, there are stable meanings attached to an event or experience that the interviewer must use his or her best endeavors to uncover. This approach fails to recognize the ambivalence characteristic of much of our thinking. Whyte points to the shortcomings of this approach:

> In dealing with subjective material, the interviewer is, of course, not trying to discover the *true attitude or sentiment* of the informant. He should recognize that ambivalence is a fairly common condition of man—that men can and do hold conflicting sentiments at any given time. Furthermore, men hold varying sentiments according to the situations in which they find themselves. (1980:117, emphasis in original)

Such ambivalence is illustrated in a recent study of mothers' understandings of health in young babies (Lauritzen 1997). Lauritzen interviewed twenty-nine mothers repeatedly during the first six months of their babies' lives. Mothers were encouraged to talk freely and the interviews revolved around issues of the babies' health and well-being. From the interview data, Lauritzen identified three basic notions of child health. First, health was something that was given or not given. Its presence or absence in a child was a matter of luck. Second, health was extremely precarious, requiring continuous preventive work by mothers. Finally, health was assumed to be a fixed resource, which the child was capable of using to cope with attacks from the environment. These three notions of health could be seen as contradictory, or at least in tension with one another. The idea that health is a matter of luck is in direct opposition to the idea that it has to be continuously worked on. Similarly the idea that a child is capable of coping with attacks from the environment is contrary to the idea that mothers need continuously to work on their babies' health. However, Lauritzen resists the temptation to allocate the mothers across these three categories. She observes that the mothers actually draw on all these categories in the course of their interviews: they "oscillate" (ibid.:444) between these different positions. Lauritzen concludes that the women's interview talk cannot be interpreted as reproducing stable health beliefs. Rather, their accounts are intertwined with their presentations of themselves as being responsible, determined and devoted mothers who do not leave the decisions to others— as "worthy" parents. (ibid.:454)

Lauritzen's analysis leads us to the second problematic assumption underpinning the claim that interview accounts can be used in a straight-forward manner to access the motivations and meanings behind the behavior of individuals. This is the assumption that the meanings and motivations expressed by informants at interview can be treated as objective represen-tations of the mental states underlying their actions. The study of benzo-diazepine use carried out by North and her colleagues and referred to above illustrates this point. Its declared aim was "to gain insights into the mean-ings that the consumption of these drugs has for their users" (North, Davis, & Powell 1995:633). In reporting their findings, the authors treat their in-formants' responses as an accurate representation of their motivations in taking these drugs. They state, for example, that "these women tended to use medication to block out fear or numb pain" (ibid.:639). Certainly this was how some of the women *presented* their drug-taking within the inter-views. North and colleagues give the example of one woman who described how she used benzodiazepines to enable her to cope with fear of an aggres-sive, heavy-drinking partner. The authors conclude that "the community-based participants were not passive recipients of benzodiazepines, and weighed up the costs, the risks of side-effects, dependence, and potential social alienation against the benefits, and most decided that benzodiaz-epines improved their quality of life" (ibid.:643).

This conclusion is not tempered by consideration of what the informants might be *doing* with their talk in the context of the interviews. This is all the more surprising since the authors themselves point out that long-standing benzodiazepine use has, at best, "borderline social legitimacy" (ibid.:646). Users are liable to face disapproval and stigmatization. The authors recognize that the fear of such negative reactions is likely to constrain the behavior and self-presentation of users. However, they do not extend this insight to their own interview data. Informants' claims and assertions are taken at face value, without considering the extent to which the interviews might be constituted as occasions for impression management.

Treating interviews as social interactions, in which all parties strive to present themselves and their behaviors to their listeners as appropriate, has radical implications. Interviews do not yield more or less adequate re-ports on mental states underlying behavior. We recognize them instead as occasions on which informants are called upon to offer "accounts" for their actions, feelings, opinions, and so on. In providing these accounts, informants seek to present themselves as competent and, indeed, moral members of their particular communities. Interviews are occasions for informants to display themselves as adequate parents, good patients, well-informed citizens, responsible adults, and competent professionals—or to produce socially acceptable explanation of their failure.

In a seminal paper, Scott and Lyman (1968) discussed the structure and content of everyday accounts. They defined an account as a "linguistic device employed whenever an action is subjected to linguistic inquiry" (ibid.:112). They argued that accounts are elicited whenever an action is subjected to evaluation of some sort and there is a suggestion that an individual may have acted inappropriately. Accounts are designed to refute such suggestions. It is not necessary for individuals to be directly challenged for them to feel called upon to produce an account. The production of accounts reflects that individual's general sensitivity to the normative context in which his or her behaviors are situated.

Clearly, interviews are occasions that are particularly likely to provoke accounts. However sensitive and nonjudgmental our interview techniques may be, they cannot be expected to neutralize informants' awareness of the ways in which their behavior could be judged and found wanting. Their responses will be constrained by the need to refute any negative evaluation that their behaviors might attract. Given the "ambivalence" and "conflicting sentiments" discussed above, which are characteristic of human action, it should not surprise us that, when asked to explain their behavior, informants offer accounts designed to rebut any suggestion that their behavior was inappropriate.

This casts a somewhat different light on the data presented by North and colleagues (North et al. 1995). We would expect informants' awareness of the "borderline legitimacy" of benzodiazepine use to shape the kinds of explanations that they offered in the interviews. The explanations offered do, indeed, attempt to rebut or defuse any negative interpretations of their behavior. For example, many informants stressed their control over their drug-taking, distancing themselves from the stereotype of "pill-rollers" (ibid.:639). They emphasized the smallness of the dose, their ability to "go without" on some occasions, and their "partial" rather than "full" dependence. They contrasted their situation with those who took escalating doses of medication, which was evidence of lack of moral fiber. Others described, in graphic detail, the intensity of their symptoms, rebutting any suggestion that their pill-taking was unwarranted self-indulgence. Some of the women pointed to the part played by others in their drug-taking. The woman discussed above who implicated her husband's drunkenness can be seen to be rebutting any suggestion that her benzodiazepine use resulted from some weakness on her own part. Her drug-taking is, rather, a very reasonable response to her husband's behavior.

Our assertion that interview talk about motivations and meanings is best treated as an account does not mean that we should assume informants are attempting to deceive us. In suggesting that the informant with the heavy-drinking spouse in North et al.'s study is producing an account, we are not questioning either her husband's drinking patterns or her consequent distress. Rather, our point is that the informant's own thinking about her benzodiazepine use is likely to be both ambivalent and complex. At a different point in time and in a different interactional context, she might well offer a range of different explanations for her drug-taking. In Chapter 2, for example, we discussed the difference between "because of" and "in order to" explanations. In the context of the interview, she is called upon to select from the possible explanations available to her. This selection will be influenced by the demands of self-presentation, and by whether the questions are looking back to evoke "because of" statements or forwards, eliciting "in order to" answers. In particular, her assumptions about normative expectations will play a significant role in the explanations that she offers for her behavior.

Should research consumers conclude that interviews can never be used to explore the meanings and motivations that lie behind behavior? Are these totally inaccessible? We think not. Our argument is that no one can simply "read off" the meanings underpinning action from interview statements. Research consumers should expect to see interview data interpreted in relation to the context of their production. Analyses should start from the question of what informants can be seen to be *doing* with their interview talk. As C. Wright Mills put it, "The reasons men give for their actions are not themselves without reasons" (1940:904). Moreover, such analysis needs to take into account the complexity, instability, and ambivalence that is characteristic of informants' understandings. This points to a third use to which interview data may be put: as a source of data on the normative context in which behavior occurs.

Displaying Moral Realities

This third approach to interview data makes a virtue of the very features of interviews that make it problematic to treat them as literal reproductions of either internal or external realities. Its starting point is the assumption that the accounts that people give in the interview situation are constrained by the need to present themselves as moral, rational, reasonable people in a context where doubts about this "hang in the air." Here what people are *doing* with their talk becomes central to the analysis rather than being treated as a source of potential bias. From this perspective interview data allow us to identify what people take to be self-evident about the world and, in particular, about the normative context in which they operate. Interview data are treated as displays of moral and cultural forms rather than as literal reports on reality. The issue of the truth or falsity of such reports is largely irrelevant within this approach. Silverman sums up this position on the legitimate use of interview data:

> research interviews offer access to a set of "moral" realities firmly located in the cultural world. Once we rid ourselves of the palpably false assumption that interview statements can stand in any simple correspondence to the real world, we can begin fruitful analysis of the real forms of representation through which they are structured. (1985:16)

Two examples from Seale (1995) will help to illustrate this approach. The first is an analysis of accounts that were given by 149 relatives, friends, and others who knew people who died alone. These were drawn from the replies that people gave to open-ended questions exploring the circumstances of the person's death, the informants' feelings about those circumstances, and the things that they might have liked to be different. Seale's informants described their shock and distress arising from their relative or friend's death alone. They stressed their eagerness to be present when the person died. Where lone deaths had occurred in hospital, accounts included reasons for the informant's absence. In some cases, absences were attributed to having followed the advice of hospital staff. In almost all cases, the informants presented their desire to be present at the death as having been thwarted. Seale interprets these accounts as demonstrating that "allowing" a friend or relative to die alone calls into question one's moral reputation. In the interviews the informants carried out moral "repair work," through which they sought to anticipate and avoid the potential charge that they had abandoned the dying person.

Central to Seale's analysis is a reading of interviews as opportunities for informants to display their moral adequacy. He makes no attempt to determine the accuracy of these accounts as reports of informants' feelings about being absent from the death. The data demonstrate the existence of strong cultural imperatives around responsibility toward the dying that challenge widely held assumptions about the denial and sequestration of death in contemporary societies. However, as Seale himself observes, treating interview data in this way does not imply that informants are free to present themselves in any way they choose. They are constrained to some extent by events outside the interview. Thus, while informants may be selective in their accounts and seek to present their behavior in a certain light, it is unlikely that the factors to which they refer have no basis in external reality.

The second example is drawn from a study by Murphy (1999, 2000) at the opposite end of the life-course. Its focus was the infant feeding practices of first-time mothers. Data were collected through repeated interviews with thirty-six mothers. A central issue was the mothers' decision whether to breast- or formula-feed their babies. This decision was made in a climate where the benefits of breast-feeding were widely canvassed. All the mothers reported receiving advice about the benefits of breast-feeding and dangers of formula-feeding from a wide range of sources, including prenatal clinics, parenting classes, and published literature. None doubted that breast-feeding was recommended as being in the best interests of the baby and as a means of protecting its short-, medium-, and long-term health. When interviewed prenatally, almost all the women declared an intention to breast-feed their babies, relating this to a commitment to offer their babies the best possible start in life. They presented their decision as evidence that they were responsible mothers intent upon doing their maternal duty. In the event, however, only six of the thirty-six women breast-fed their babies for the minimum recommended period. The others introduced formula milk at some point during the babies' first few months. Given these women's construction of breast-feeding as a maternal duty in the prenatal interviews, this meant that two-thirds of the mothers in the study fed their babies in ways that directly contradicted the ideals that they themselves had set for responsible mothers.

Murphy's analysis focused on the reasons that women offered for their decision to introduce formula milk. Like Seale, she did not concern herself with whether the reasons given accurately represented the motivation of the women at the point when they introduced formula milk. She assumed that the decision to introduce formula milk was likely to have been made at the intersection of a range of different factors and to have been characterized by a degree of ambivalence and instability. Rather, the reasons given were analyzed in terms of the normative context in which mothers feed their babies and the kinds of control to which such feeding is subject. She demonstrated that mothers' interview talk in defense of the introduction of formula could be heard as attempts to bridge the gap between their own behavior and the "ideal of the autonomous, self-reliant, prudent woman who suppresses her own needs and adopts a calculative attitude to her baby's well-being in the light of expert advice" (ibid.:318).

Both these studies illustrate the potential of interview data to extend our understanding of the social and cultural context in which health-related behaviors and interactions occur. However, the relevance of this approach is not limited to examining patient or client behaviors. It could equally well be applied to the analysis of interview data from health care providers. Allen's (1997) study, discussed above, points the way toward this kind of analysis of the interview talk of health professionals and managers. Similarly, Norris's (2001) analysis of interviews with a range of practitioners who treat musculoskeletal disorders is concerned with the rhetorical strategies that are used by individual practitioners to establish and maintain occupational boundaries between their work and that of other practitioners.

INTERACTIONAL EVENTS

The final, and probably least common, use of interview data is to study interviews as interactional events. Here the focus is not upon the content of interview talk but rather upon the way in which the interview proceeds. In other words, we are no longer concerned with *what* people say in interviews but with the interviews as a proxy for natural conversations. This approach to interview data draws upon many of the insights from conversation analysis, which was discussed in the previous chapter. Again, an example may help to clarify this approach.

Manzo and colleagues (Manzo, Blonder, & Burns 1995) carried out interviews with twenty-two people, fourteen of whom had suffered a stroke and eight who had non-stroke-related impairments. The latter were used as controls in this study. All informants were interviewed at home, in the presence of their spouses. The reported data were derived from the exchanges that followed an opening question in which informants were asked to talk about their stroke, how it happened, and how they knew they were having a stroke. The analysis does not deal with the content of these stories but looks at the ways in which the patients' spouses participated in telling the patients' stories. The authors report significant and sustained differences between the roles that the spouses of stroke victims played in the interviews and those played by the spouses of informants with non-stroke-related impairments. Compared to the control group, the stroke victims' part in relating the experience of their own illness was systematically reduced as their spouses participated more fully in the storytelling than would be expected. Manzo and colleagues document the conversational devices associated with this phenomenon. For example, stroke victims often sought to elicit their spouse's approval for their narrative with tag questions (e.g., "Didn't I?" "Isn't that right?"). Spouses engaged in competitive storytelling, supplementing, correcting, or contradicting stories told by stroke victims. They sometimes answered questions directed at the patients and reissued questions that the interviewer had asked of the patients. These phenomena were found in interviews with the stroke patients, irrespective of whether they were linguistically impaired as a result of the stroke. By contrast, none of these features were observed in interviews with nonstroke patients where the spouses only participated when specifically invited to do so by either the interviewer or the patient.

These researchers did not use these interviews to elicit a report of either the patients' experiences or of external reality. These interviews were treated as a proxy for naturally occurring conversations. The analytic focus is upon the way in which the interview talk is organized. The authors use this to explore the social and interactional consequences of stroke and, in particular, the way in which patients' ability to tell their own stories was severely compromised not only as a result of stroke-related neurological deficits but also of interactional patterns that undermined their capacity to speak for themselves.

CONCLUSION

In this chapter we have argued that qualitative interviews can make a significant contribution to health studies. At times, such interviews may be the method of choice. They can provide data on settings and social processes that would not otherwise be open to investigation. This may be because the phenomenon we are interested in does not occur in a focused and identifiable location that would permit observation. Alternatively, it may occur in a setting that is private or one to which access is blocked. Qualitative research interviews can also offer an escape route from some of the more intransigent problems and contradictions that beset quantitative forms of interviewing. The data they elicit can undermine the taken-for-granted assumptions of researchers and policymakers. In doing so, they offer the opportunity to discover aspects of a policy-relevant issue or problem that could not have been predicted at the outset of a study and the flexibility to pursue these leads once identified.

Nevertheless, the potential of qualitative interviews will not be fully exploited unless researchers take a sophisticated approach to the analysis of their data. When interviews are used to generate reports on external realities, such an approach implies a conscientious and explicit assessment of the trustworthiness of the data obtained. Where they are used to elicit accounts of informants' internal realities, then analysis needs to be sensitive to the interactional and political contexts in which the data were generated. In this way researchers will guard against drawing facile conclusions about the motives and meanings of health care providers and recipients on the basis of interview statements.

NOTES

1. Qualitative researchers tend to describe the people they interview as "informants" rather than "respondents" or "interviewees." This stresses the more active role that they are thought to play in the research—they do not merely *respond* to the researcher's questions but they *inform* the researcher about themselves and their experiences.

2. Some of the difficulties that qualitative research proposals encounter with IRBs are discussed in Chapter 8.

3. An experimental demonstration of this can be found in McHugh (1968). Students were told that they were participating in a trial of a new form of counseling where they would have to ask advice from a counselor hidden behind a screen, who would only answer "yes" or "no" to their questions. The counselor generated the answers at random while McHugh recorded the students' reflections. Despite the limited information available to them and the occasionally inconsistent answers they received, the student participants had no difficulty in finding the experience to have been sensible, meaningful, and even helpful. However, what each student took from the encounter depended entirely on what he or she had brought to it.

4. Macintyre's (1978) study of obstetric clerking, which we cited in the previous chapter, is, of course, another example of this phenomenon, although in that context the interviewers were preemptively answering the problematic questions.

6

Selection and Sampling in Qualitative Research

In Chapter 3 we considered the range of purposes to which health-related qualitative research might profitably be applied. These included the production of rigorous descriptions of both formal and informal dimensions of health care practice and organization, uncovering the dynamic processes underlying particular outcomes, the discovery of unanticipated but relevant dimensions to a problem, and the study of the interaction between interventions and context. In translating these broad purposes into a research design, researchers quickly confront the question of whom or what to study. As in all research, it is rarely possible for qualitative researchers to examine every case of the phenomenon in which they are interested. Rather they are obliged to select some cases from the population of those that conceivably might be of interest. Such selection decisions are highly consequential for the usefulness of research findings to policymakers.

It is relatively rare, though not unheard of, for policymakers and practitioners to be interested primarily in the specific cases studied by researchers. If the phenomenon under study is sufficiently significant then it may be worth studying for its own sake (Seale 1999). More usually, however, research users are concerned about what studying particular settings or individuals can tell us about phenomena of more general relevance. The requirement for findings of general relevance raises some important questions about qualitative research. Can the significance or utility of a research study extend beyond the case or cases actually studied? Is it possible for qualitative researchers to produce findings of more than local significance? Is qualitative research restricted to producing anecdotal accounts that, however interesting, have indeterminate relevance beyond the particular settings in which they were produced?

GENERALIZABILITY IN QUALITATIVE RESEARCH

Some qualitative researchers dismiss generalizability as either inappropriate or unobtainable in qualitative research. For example, Merriam argues that qualitative research should not be concerned with drawing conclusions that extend beyond the cases actually studied:

> One selects a case study approach because one wishes to understand the particular in depth, not because one wishes to know what is generally true of the many. (1988:173)

Similarly, Stake suggests that while some generalization may be possible from studies of particular cases, this is not the primary goal of such research. The real object should be "particularization" rather than generalization:

> We take a particular case and come to know it well, not primarily as to how it is different from others but what it is, what it does. There is an emphasis upon uniqueness, and that implies knowledge of others that the case is different from, but the emphasis is upon understanding the case itself. (1995:8)

By contrast, we believe that, in most cases where one is seeking to carry out research to inform policy and practice, a central concern should be with the light that the close investigation of settings or individuals can thrown on other, comparable individuals or settings (Schofield 1993). In the first chapter of this book we addressed arguments about the scientific status of qualitative research. We argued that policy-relevant qualitative research both can and should aspire to be scientific. Generalizability is often, and in our view quite rightly, taken to be one of the hallmarks of science (Smith 1975). In this chapter, we turn to consider the potential of qualitative research for meeting this criterion. Attempts to generalize beyond the data obtained immediately raise questions about the methods used to select the setting(s) or people studied.

PROBABILITY SAMPLING AND QUALITATIVE RESEARCH

Within quantitative research traditions, generalizability is normally pursued via sample-to-population inference, using the techniques of probabilistic statistics. The use of such techniques allows us to estimate, within precise margins of error, the distribution of a phenomenon in the universe from which it is drawn. They are an effective means of dealing with the problem that arises when the universe of interest is too large for us to study it in its entirety. Such techniques depend, among other things, upon achieving an adequate sample size to satisfy the assumptions of the methods being used. As we have seen in previous chapters, qualitative observational research is frequently carried out in a single setting or, at best, in a small number of settings. Similarly, qualitative interview studies are generally restricted to relatively small sample sizes. The ratio of settings or individuals studied to the number in the aggregate is usually too low to allow statistical inference (Hammersley 1992f). As a result, qualitative research studies rarely meet the assumptions of probabilistic sampling methods, making the use of such methods impractical.

There is, however, nothing in the logic of qualitative research that restricts it to the small sample sizes that make statistically based sample-to-population inference impossible. The problem is a practical rather than a conceptual one. Given sufficient resources and unlimited research access, it would be perfectly possible for observational studies to be carried out in large numbers of randomly selected settings. Similarly, qualitative interview studies with randomly selected informants, which are sufficiently large to permit statistical analysis, are, in principle, possible. However, the time-consuming data collection and analysis, which are characteristic of qualitative research, mean that it is unusual for sufficient resources to be available to permit the collection of data that would allow statistical inference from sample to population.

The use of nonprobability sampling methods in qualitative research is best seen as a pragmatic compromise between breadth and depth. The various contributions that qualitative research can make to the evidence base of health care policy and practice arise largely from the in-depth nature of qualitative research. Neither identifying routine but unnoticed aspects of organizational life, nor uncovering the processes that underlie observed outcomes, nor the interplay between activities and the context in which they occur, are features of health care settings that are amenable to superficial investigation. They demand lengthy periods of fieldwork and/ or interviewing. The data generated do not lend themselves to routinized categorization or analysis. Qualitative research is irreducibly labor intensive and inevitably time consuming. One practical consequence of this is that qualitative researchers rarely find themselves in a position where they can combine, in the same study, the depth that is the great strength of their methods with the breadth that is afforded through the use of probability sampling techniques. Given a forced choice, qualitative researchers tend to opt for depth rather than breadth.

Such pragmatic choices are not, of course, the sole preserve of qualitative researchers. It is relatively unusual, even in quantitative research, for statistical generalization to the population of interest to be fully warranted (Bryman 1988). One of the problems, which is shared by both qualitative and quantitative researchers, is that the populations in which they are interested are rarely fully itemized (Firestone 1993). As a consequence, re-searchers are often obliged to treat a group that they can itemize as a proxy for the population that they cannot. The result is that, while statistical samples may be representative of the particular group from which they have been drawn, they are rarely representative of the population to which research consumers might wish to generalize.

COMBINING PRINCIPLE AND PRAGMATISM
IN QUALITATIVE RESEARCH

The practical difficulties associated with using probability sampling in qualitative research do not, however, oblige us to abandon a commitment to generalizability or to be guided in our sampling decisions by nothing more than opportunism. This is not to say that opportunism has no role to play in qualitative research. In some cases, particularly where the phenom-enon of interest is highly sensitive or illicit, or the relevant population is mobile or known to be reluctant to participate in research, opportunistic sampling may be the only avenue open to a researcher. Again, where, for example, a researcher wishes to combine intensive fieldwork in an emer-gency room or an intensive care unit with other responsibilities such as clinical work or teaching students, the only option may be to carry out most of the data collection in an institution close to his or her place of employ-ment. Similarly, opportunistic approaches to sampling may be justifiable in the initial, exploratory phases of a research study. However, those who are committed to striving for cumulative knowledge, to inform policy and practice in health care, will be reluctant to settle for mere opportunism in selecting the objects of study. If we reject the notion that such knowledge is merely a mosaic of multiple slices of life that can be juxtaposed with one another (see Denzin 1983) we shall treat opportunistic sampling as a method of last resort in anything other than the most preliminary and ex-ploratory research studies.

Pragmatism is not, however, entirely irrelevant to sampling decisions. Just as in quantitative research, sample selection in qualitative studies is the art of the possible. However elegant a sampling design may be, it will be useless if limited research funds make it impractical or if it is impossible to gain access to the settings or groups selected. Rather we suggest that, in selection decisions, pragmatic considerations should be integrated with a commitment to drawing samples in a systematic and principled way (Schofield 1993). As we shall see below, the particular principles underly-ing such decisions will depend upon the goals and priorities of a particu-lar study.

This interplay between pragmatism and principle is well-illustrated in

Edgerton's (1967) classic study of the management of stigma by "mentally retarded people". For practical reasons, Edgerton was obliged to restrict his study to a single research site. This is, of course, similar to many clinical trials where the effectiveness of an intervention is investigated in a small number of settings, leaving the generalizability of findings to other settings open to question. However, as in quantitative research, we need to distinguish between difficulties in generalizing beyond the population studied and the extent to which it is valid to generalize from the individuals or events studied within a local setting to the universe of individuals or events present within that setting. In the latter case, we are particularly concerned with the risk that the way in which a sample is drawn within a setting distorts the findings from the research. As in experimental research, the imperative is for clear information about how the sample was selected to be made available so that such sources of potential bias or atypicality can be identified.

A clear statement of the selection criteria used allows us to identify the characteristics of those to whom generalization is, at least in principle, possible. Edgerton's study remains a model in this respect. It focussed on the ways in which mentally retarded people—to use the contemporary terminology—managed their lives and perceived themselves, when discharged from institutional care and left to their own devices in a large city. The setting most readily available for the study was "Pacific State Hospital," a large state institution in California. However, within the population of people with a diagnosis of mental retardation attached in some way to this hospital, decisions about whom to study still had to be made. Edgerton identified explicit criteria that his sample would need to meet to enable him to investigate this topic:

> In order to select persons who had a reasonable chance of success in independent city living, persons would have to be selected who were near the upper limits of the mildly retarded range, both in terms of their measured IQs and their estimated social competence. These persons also needed to have been discharged from the hospital and to have remained free from any formal supervision either by Pacific State Hospital or any other social agency or institution. Finally, at the time of their release, these persons must have been free from any formal supervision or guardianship of parents, relatives or friends; they must have been released with the explicit understanding that they were expected to live on their own resources. (ibid.:10)

By clarifying the basis of selection within the setting in this way, Edgerton enables the reader to identify the population to which his findings might, potentially at least, be generalized. However, as Edgerton explained, the relevance of findings from this study could well extend beyond

those who were diagnosed as being at the upper limits of the mildly retarded range. In effect, Edgerton argues that they could be seen as a test
case:

> If there were any group of persons once institutionalized as being mentally
> retarded who could be expected to have an opportunity for successful inde-
> pendent living outside an institution, it would be this group. (ibid.:11)

In other words, Edgerton had good theoretical reasons for the criteria
he adopted, even though the resultant sample was, by definition, atypical of all those who were institutionalized with a diagnosis of mental
retardation.

Edgerton then went on to identify a cohort of ex-patients from Pacific
State Hospital who met the criteria stipulated. These were the graduates
from one of the hospital's training and rehabilitation programs who had
been discharged from the hospital without any reservations on their freedom, in a ten-year period. Patients selected for this program had fallen into
the upper stratum of the hospital's mildly retarded patients, with regard
to their IQs, their demonstrated social competence, and their demonstrated
emotional stability.

One hundred and ten ex-patients who had graduated from the program
in the specified period were identified. Edgerton then undertook an ener-
getic search for all these ex-patients and within twelve months he had located all but twelve of the original number. He then compared certain
characteristics (such as IQ, age, and date of discharge) of the twelve people
who were not traced with those of the remaining ninety-eight who were.
There was no substantial variation in these characteristics between those
who had been contacted and those who had not.

At this point, practical considerations again constrained the selection
process. Many of the former patients had migrated long distances from the
hospital. Since Edgerton was proposing to carry out extensive fieldwork,
including long and repeated interviews and participant observation of the
lives of the former patients, the cost of including all these patients in the
study would have been prohibitive. He therefore decided to limit the study
to the fifty-three ex-patients who lived within a fifty-mile radius of the
hospital. Once again, he compared the basic descriptive data concerning
members of the cohort who remained inside the fifty-mile radius study area
and those who did not and found that, other than mobility, there were no
major differences.

Edgerton's study is an excellent example of the way in which it is possible to combine principle and pragmatism in sampling decisions in qualitative research. In this particular case, the primary consideration was
theoretical. He identified a subgroup of people who had been institution-

alized with mental retardation and who were relevant to the objectives of his study. Having done so, a second principle—that of typicality was introduced. Edgerton wanted to ensure that, as far as possible, the people included in his study were typical of all those in the cohort who had met the theoretical criteria. Throughout the process, Edgerton combined these principled selection decisions with a pragmatic concern to complete the study within the resources available.

ENHANCING THE TYPICALITY OF QUALITATIVE RESEARCH

Qualitative researchers, and the policymakers and practitioners who use their findings, are frequently concerned about the typicality of findings and the possibility of using such findings as the basis for empirical generalizations. We have already discussed some of the difficulties of using probability sampling methods in qualitative research. However, these difficulties do not prevent us from making reasonable judgments about the representativeness or typicality of findings from a research study (Hammersley 1992f). As Hammersley suggests, there are a number of sources of information that can inform judgments about the potential generalizability of research findings.

For example, it is possible to use published statistics to inform the sampling design of a qualitative study. This can be particularly useful where the intensive nature of a qualitative research study limits the sample size. In the interview study of the choices that mothers make about how to feed their babies, which was introduced in the previous chapter, Murphy (1999, 2000) followed a cohort of first-time mothers from late pregnancy until their babies' second birthdays. In addition to six interviews with each mother, data were also collected from the mothers' partners, other members of their social networks, and the health professionals who advised them about infant feeding. The scope of the data collection and analysis meant that the size of the main sample had to be restricted to thirty-six mothers. Even with this relatively small sample, more than three hundred interviews, each lasting at least one hour, were carried out. It was clear that, with a sample of this size, the risk of selecting an atypical group of participants was considerable. Murphy sought to minimize this risk by drawing on the findings of large-scale surveys of U.K. infant feeding practices (White, Freeth, & O'Brien 1992; Foster, Lader, & Cheesbrough 1997). These studies had shown that infant feeding practices varied with both occupational class and the age of the mother. A quota sample was devised to avoid overrepresenting women in particular occupational classes or age groups. Twelve mothers were recruited from higher occupational classes, twelve from intermediate occupational classes, and twelve from lower occupational classes. Half the women in each occupational grouping were below the mean age at birth of first baby for that grouping, and half were above. The quota was filled by sequentially drawn women from the birth registers of ten general medical practices within a ten-mile radius of one U.K. city with recruitment continuing until the quotas were filled.

Clearly, there are limitations to the extent to which this kind of quota sampling can ensure generalizability. The findings from such research cannot lay claim to the representativeness that probability sampling offers. Nor was it possible to incorporate all the variables that have been identified or might be identified as related to infant feeding practices into the quota design. Nevertheless, by drawing upon the findings from large-scale surveys, it was possible to avoid two major sources of atypicality. The usefulness of this approach was underscored when the distribution of infant feeding practices reported by the women in the study was found to reflect those reported in the large-scale surveys.

Qualitative researchers may also seek to increase the typicality of their sample by excluding cases that are atypical in particular ways. For example, in a well-known qualitative study, Fred Davis (1963) explored the impact of polio on fourteen children and their families. The study design was longitudinal and involved repeated contacts with the child, the child's parents, and the relevant hospital personnel. It resulted in what Davis describes as a "voluminous body of interview, observational, test and medical data" (ibid.:181), including an average of fifty hours of interviewing with each family. This is again an instance where the researchers have opted to trade the breadth of data that might have been generated from a larger sample for the depth that comes from the detailed study of a small number of cases.

Davis explains that the sample was designed "to ensure a certain degree of homogeneity among cases and representativeness with respect to the major pathological and epidemiological characteristics of the disease" (ibid.:182). In practice this meant that, since 65 percent of the children affected by polio in the area in which he was working were aged between four and twelve years of age, Davis restricted his sample to this age group. Likewise, since 70 percent of children had the most common form of polio (paralytic polio), he excluded those with the less common bulbar and encephalitic forms. This kind of homogeneous sample does have the advantage of setting some boundaries to the informal generalizations that might be drawn from the study. It warns the reader against assuming that the findings would be equally relevant to families where an infant or teenager contracted the disease. However, it can also raise some complex political and ethical issues particularly about the exclusion of minority groups from research. In the case of Davis's research, nonwhite children and those not judged to have come from "clinically normal" homes were excluded. In this case the definition of "clinically normal" home included the requirement that the child's mother be present. This research was carried out half a century ago and it is unlikely that these kinds of exclusion criteria, or the rationales offered to justify them, would be considered acceptable today. However, this study is a useful reminder that selection decisions directed toward avoiding atypicality always involve value judgments about which variables should be treated as relevant or irrelevant to judgments of what constitutes typicality.

A further strategy for enhancing the claims to typicality of qualitative research projects involves coordinating a number of qualitative studies so that it is possible to cover a wider range of naturally occurring variation than would be possible in a single study. In some cases, this is achieved through different researchers cooperating to study different aspects of the same phenomenon. For example, Miller and Silverman (1995) collaborated across their separate studies of how people talk about troubles in counseling settings. Silverman's study was carried out in a British hemophilia center where counseling was delivered to people who were HIV-positive. Miller's data were collected in a U.S. family therapy center. The two researchers developed a comparative analysis, which focused upon the similarities in three elements of counselor-client interaction (trouble definitions, trouble remedies, and the social contexts of clients' troubles) that were identified in both settings.

A variation on this strategy is for researchers to carry out intensive fieldwork in one or more settings and then to investigate the typicality of their findings through shorter periods of study in other parallel or similar settings. This was the approach adopted by Guillemin and Holmstrom (1986) in their study of decision-making in intensive care nurseries, which was discussed in Chapters 2 and 3. The researchers carried out the bulk of their fieldwork in the intensive care nursery of just one hospital (Northeast Pacific). They spent six months attending interdisciplinary rounds, seminars, conferences, and discussions in that hospital and then conducted an eight-month period of observation there. Having completed their research at Northeast Pacific, they then embarked on a series of site visits to other intensive care nurseries. They describe the purpose of these visits as "to test our observations at Northeast Pacific and to gain a comparative perspective on national and international variations in neonatal care" (ibid.:19).

They were unable to carry out the same level of intensive fieldwork in these other hospitals but by interviewing the staff in fourteen newborn intensive care units in the United States and comparable nurseries in England, the Netherlands, East and West Germany, France, and Brazil, they were able to examine the generalizability of the findings from their initial case study.

We have discussed a number of strategies that qualitative researchers may adopt to enhance the generalizability of their research findings. None of these strategies will guarantee the typicality of the settings or individuals studied. In keeping with the overall perspective that we have adopted in this book, they may be best seen as the means by which error can be limited (see Chapters 1 and 9). The responsibility for deciding the extent to which it is reasonable to draw general conclusions from the findings of a particular study will, in the end, always be invested in the reader of research reports. Such decisions will always be a matter of judgment. As Seale (1999) points out, judgments of this kind always involve a good deal of common sense on the part of research consumers in deciding whether the context in which the research was carried out is sufficiently similar to the context in which one is proposing to apply its finding to make them relevant to the new situation. The ability of the reader to make such judgments is highly dependent upon the information researchers make available about the individuals, groups, or settings studied. We pursue this issue in Chapter 9 when we consider the criteria for evaluating qualitative research studies.

SAMPLING TO DEVELOP AND TEST THEORY

It is important to note that the search for typicality is not always either the only or the primary purpose that underlies selection decisions in qualitative research. Strategic selection decisions can also, for example, enable researchers to examine tentative hypotheses drawn from earlier work or test out some of the researchers' own prior assumptions. For example, in a recent study of lay beliefs about heart disease, Carol Emslie and her colleagues carried out sixty-one qualitative interviews with men and women in the west of Scotland (Emslie, Hunt, & Watt 2001; Hunt, Emslie, & Watt 2000). For the purposes of this study, they drew a subsample from a cross-sectional survey of cardiorespiratory disease, which was conducted in 1996 in the west of Scotland. The researchers had several objectives, which were reflected in their sampling strategy. First, they wanted to examine lay notions of "family history" of heart disease. Since it seemed possible that such notions would be related in some way to informants' own family experiences of heart disease, they selected half of their sample from respondents to the 1996 survey who reported that heart problems "ran in their family" and half from those who did not. They also wanted to establish whether lay perceptions of heart problems varied by social class and by gender. They therefore ensured that half their sample was male and half was female and contained similar numbers of informants from socially nonmobile (i.e., both informants and their fathers in same occupational class) manual and nonmanual occupations. These sampling decisions ensured that the researchers were able to carry out the kinds of comparative analysis of their data that enabled them to examine the tentative hypotheses underlying their research design.

The approach adopted by Emslie and her colleagues is a form of theoretical sampling (Glaser & Strauss 1967). The primary purpose of their selection strategy was to draw a sample that was a suitable vehicle for examining the theoretical propositions relevant to their study. Emerson defines theoretical sampling as a procedure "in which new observations are explicitly to pursue analytically relevant distinctions rather than to establish the frequency or distribution of phenomena" (1981:360).

There is some confusion about what can be achieved through theoretical sampling. As both Hammersley (1992f) and Seale (1999) have observed, some people have suggested that theoretical sampling is a means by which the truth or falsity of universal deterministic laws of human or social behavior could be established. This position presupposes the existence of such universal laws and the associated belief that human behavior is fully causally determined. Relatively few social scientists would subscribe to this or what we might describe as the strong program of using theoretical sampling as a means of establishing such universal claims. The subtle realist position may be better described as one based on empirical generalization, where theories are collections of second-level descriptions, recasting the specifics of particular cases into a more abstract language that makes them potentially transferable to the analysis of other cases. We shall return to this concept of theory in Chapter 7.

Theoretical sampling should be understood as a process by which the researcher sets critical tests for the general validity of hypotheses and seeks to establish the conditions under which they do or do not hold (Dingwall 1992). As such, it is integral to the pursuit of a cumulative body of knowledge by empirical generalization through qualitative research. The object is to establish whether some process or phenomenon that is identified in a specified setting can or cannot also be found in other settings that are similar or different in some specified way.

Theoretical sampling involves selecting cases (whether observational settings or documentary materials or interview informants) that will act as critical tests of the limits of the propositions arising out of previous research. It can be used to select the initial focus and/or setting for a particular study. Buckholdt and Gubrium's (1979) study of the operation of an institution for the treatment of emotionally disturbed young people is an example of this kind of approach. Gubrium (1975) had previously conducted research in an American nursing home. From the findings of this observational study, he had concluded that "senility" was "a useful and/or required way of reading aged patients' behavior in nursing homes as well as a description of the mental status of select patients" (Buckholdt &

Gubrium 1979:249). These findings were consistent with a more general hypothesis that

> whatever people appear to be as patients or clients in institutions like nursing homes, psychiatric hospitals, and residential treatment centers, their status is as much an artifact of how features of their lives are read and defined as an artifact of the features themselves. (ibid.)

This hypothesis extends beyond the bounded phenomenon of senility in nursing homes that Gubrium had originally investigated. It involves a claim that a social process observed in one setting is of more general relevance to all institutions in which some form of "caretaking" takes place. In effect a more abstract hypothesis is tentatively derived from a specific phenomenon observed in a particular kind of setting.

To test the validity of this more general hypothesis, Buckholdt and Gubrium planned to carry out an empirical investigation of a somewhat different institution. They developed a "wish-list" detailing the features that would characterize the institution to be investigated next:

> Required was a human service institution with an official goal of treating clients for their problems. This eliminated the kind of services that primarily involved client placement and transfer, the function of many public welfare agencies. We needed a field site where treatment was conducted, preferably on a full-time basis with full-time clients. Nursing homes, mental hospitals and residential treatment centers met this requirement. Since our focus was to be treatment practice, it was important the field site selected not only have treatment as a goal but have an ongoing treatment program. Compared to a number of institutions, Cedarview [the institution finally selected] had an extensive multidisciplinary program with more of the same in the works. Moreover, it was important to select the best institution of its kind (based on conventional criteria) in order to minimize questions that might arise over our interpretations, questions suggesting our findings were not general ones but the result of professional staff members' shortcomings. Again Cedarview fulfilled this requirement, according to local public welfare officials and other human service pundits. (ibid.:250)

By choosing to study a facility for the treatment of young people, Buckholdt and Gubrium set a particularly tough test of the general relevance of findings derived from the study of nursing homes that catered largely for elderly people. They were concerned to test out the empirical validity of their claim that "not only does people's care status flow with their caretakers' practices, but that this happens at all points of the life-course" (ibid.:250).

Other studies in which theoretical considerations have informed initial sampling decisions include Bosk's (1979) research on the management of medical failure, Wiener's (2000) study of accountability in U.S. hospitals (both of which were discussed in previous chapters) and Timmermans's (1999) investigation of the use of cardiopulmonary resuscitation in U.S. emergency departments, which is taken up in Chapter 8. In each case, the researchers made initial sampling decisions that were informed by theoretical assumptions about likely sources of contrast between different kinds of facility.

Bosk carried out his study in the surgical department of one hospital. Four surgical services operated within this hospital and Bosk elected to study two of these in depth. He explains the thinking behind his selection decision and its consequences:

> These two different services were chosen by the logic of the constant comparative method (Glaser & Strauss 1967). The general surgical services at Pacific Hospital varied in their approach to surgical work along a continuum, the poles of which were low clinical-high research orientation and high clinical-low research orientation ... the two attendings for Able Service ... run the service from a distance. The two surgeons spend more time involved in their research activity than they do in direct clinical care of their patients. ... The two attendings on the Baker Service ... spend more time involved in direct patient care. ... The Baker Service is busier than the Able Service. ... I made an initial assumption that was incorrect in a way that proved serendipitous. I assumed that, both because of the different leadership styles of the Able and Baker attendings and because of the different emphases of their services, I would have a natural comparison of the ways errors were detected, coded and redressed in two different social groups, while holding the task constant. However, no interactionally significant differences emerged between the Able and Baker Services in the handling of errors. ... This alerted me to an underlying uniformity that informed the surgical world view and I began to specify what the elements that accounted for that uniformity were and how when taken together they formed a unique *gestalt*. (Bosk 1979:8–13)

Similar theoretical considerations are clearly present (though not quite so clearly explicated) in both Wiener's and Timmermans's studies. Most of Wiener's fieldwork was carried out in two hospitals in contrasting locations and which served very different populations. One was a 344-bed hospital in a large metropolitan area that served a lower-economic population characterized by cultural diversity. The other was a 438-bed hospital in a suburban community that served a largely middle-class population. The selection of these two hospitals appears to reflect an assumption that the processes Wiener is concerned with could well differ according to the location and population served. Similarly, Timmermans elected to carry out his fieldwork in two contrasting emergency departments. One of these was a level-one trauma center with a trauma surgeon, neurosurgeon, and cardiac surgeon constantly on call. The other was in a level-two trauma center with less stringent staffing requirements and more limited services. Again the assumption underpinning this selection decision appears to be that the level of staffing and services might be expected to have an impact on the practices surrounding cardiopulmonary resuscitation.

As we saw in Bosk's study of surgical errors, this kind of theoretical sampling opens up possibilities for theoretical refinement irrespective of whether the anticipated contrasts are found in the subsequent data. Where differences are found between contrasting settings, this can point to significant dimensions of the phenomenon under study. Where no differences are found, this enhances our confidence that the relevance of the findings extends beyond those facilities or institutions that share the narrowly defined characteristics of the particular setting(s) studied.

SAMPLING DECISIONS DURING A QUALITATIVE RESEARCH STUDY

Theoretical sampling is not a process that is confined to the initial stages of qualitative research. As discussed in Chapter 3, one of the strengths of qualitative research lies in the opportunity it affords for flexible examination of concepts and hypotheses that emerge in the course of the research itself. In qualitative research, sampling decisions recur throughout the research process. In the early stages of the research, the investigator's observations will form the basis of some preliminary and somewhat tentative hypotheses. Further decisions then have to be made about how these emergent ideas could be tested out through further data collection and analysis. Glaser and Strauss argued that, in qualitative research, "the active search for data occurs as the researcher asks himself the next theoretically relevant question, which in turn, directs him to seek particular groups for study" (1967:59). They provide a detailed account of how this process operated during the fieldwork for their book *Awareness of Dying* (Glaser & Strauss 1965b):

> Visits to the various medical services were scheduled as follows: I wished first to look at services that minimized patient awareness (and so looked first at a premature baby service and then at a neurosurgical service where patients were frequently comatose). I wished next to look at dying in a situation where expectancy of staff and often patients was great and dying was quick, so I observed on an Intensive Care Unit. Then I wished to observe on a service where staff expectations of terminality were great but where the patient's might or might not be, and where dying tended to be slow. So I looked next at a cancer service. I wished then to look at conditions where death was unexpected and rapid, and so looked at an emergency service. While we were looking at some different types of services, we also observed the above types

of service at other types of hospitals. So our scheduling of types of service was directed by a general conceptual scheme—which included hypotheses about awareness, expectedness and rate of dying—as well as by a developing conceptual structure including matters not at first envisioned. Sometimes we returned to services after the initial two or three or four weeks of continuous observation, in order to check upon items which needed checking or had been missed in the initial period. (Glaser & Strauss 1967:59)

Bosk's account of the way in which he conducted the fieldwork for his study of surgical mistakes indicates a similar iterative relationship between the emergent analysis and decisions about future data collection:

For two to three months I would be totally immersed in fieldwork; I would go to the hospital six days a week and stay the course of the day. Notes were taken as soon after events as possible, routinely within twenty-four hours. Field notes attempted to record events in as narrative or straightforward fashion as possible. Then, after this intense immersion, I would leave the field for two weeks to a month and perform and *"in situ"* analysis on my field notes. I developed categories, interpretations, and hypotheses from the field notes and discovered where my data were weak and where my observations needed to be concentrated in the future. I then returned to the field for further observation. In this way I "saturated" my categories and "grounded" my theory (Glaser & Strauss 1967). I left the field only when my observations had reached the point of diminishing marginal utility. (1979:14–15)

Hammersley and Atkinson refer to sampling decisions that are internal to a particular study as "sampling within the case" (1995:45):

Decisions must be made about where to observe and when, who to talk to and what to ask, as well as what to record and how. In this process we are not only deciding what is and what is not relevant to the case under study but also usually sampling from the data available in the case. (ibid.:46)

Some of these "within case" sampling decisions will involve ensuring that observations made at one time period hold good at another. Health care facilities commonly have strong diurnal and seasonal rhythms. Some periods are busier than others. One might expect behavior and interactions to vary according to the time of day and the time of year. Researchers are therefore concerned to avoid limiting their observations in ways that might mislead them into assuming that practices observed at one period have more general significance than they actually do. Fieldwork is often designed to avoid this danger. For example, Guillemin and Holmstrom (1986) describe how they made a point of being at the neonatal intensive care unit they studied for much of the working day and in the evenings, including after family visits were over, when the staff were able to relax. Similarly,

Timmermans (1999) sought to ensure that he was present at emergency resuscitations in the emergency room he was studying, irrespective of when they occurred. To achieve this, he arranged to be included in the hospital's automatic paging system whenever the hospital was notified of an impending admission by the ambulance service.

"Within case" sampling often also involves ensuring that the full range of people present in a setting is adequately represented in the data collected. In most settings there are some informants with whom it is easier to establish a relationship than others. Renee Anspach (1993) describes how, initially at least, it was difficult to establish more than the most rudimentary relationships with the staff in the intensive care nursery she was observing. She compares the nursery to a "closed society" and describes the efforts she went to in the early months of her study to establish working relationships with the staff. Some staff took a special interest in the study and provided exceptionally candid accounts of the politics of the nursery and their views of the life-and-death decisions. However, as Anspach fully recognized, restricting her data collection to those informants who were sympathetic to her study, risked producing research findings that were highly unrepresentative of the other staff in the setting:

> For several reasons, of course, my research design required me to go beyond a few informants and to cultivate research relationships with a larger and more diverse group of staff members. First, I needed a representative sense of the various viewpoints that were called into play in a given decision. I also needed a more diverse set of informants to provide information about the organization of the nursery and to provide multiple accounts of decisions I would inevitably miss. (ibid.:186)

Sampling within the case is an important means by which qualitative researchers can expose their emerging analyses to the possibility of contradiction. The danger of overgeneralization from a relatively small corpus of data is ever-present in qualitative research. A deliberate and conscientious search for negative or deviant cases is an important strategy for avoiding this kind of mistake. This is an issue to which we shall return in Chapter 9, when we consider the various criteria that we might apply in judging the quality of qualitative research.

CONCLUSION

The focus of this chapter has been on the issues of selection and sampling in relation to qualitative research. We have argued that it is rarely feasible to combine the intensive data collection and analysis characteristic of qualitative research with the procedures of probability sampling. This means that most qualitative studies are unable to make the kinds of robust claims to statistical representativeness that such procedures allow. Typically, qualitative researchers attach greater weight to other aspects of research design. However, this does not mean that qualitative researcher should simply abandon the aspiration to produce findings that are of more than local relevance. In this chapter, we have discussed some of the approaches that such researchers employ as they adopt a strategic and principled approach to the selection of informants and settings through which to pursue the objectives of their research. These are of utmost significance to commissioners who are making research funding decisions and to research consumers as they assess the relevance of findings from qualitative research to the settings or settings for which they are responsible.

7

The Analysis of Qualitative Data

Qualitative research can easily generate data that are, in the words of Bryman and Burgess, "voluminous, unstructured and unwieldy" (1994:216). This is not inevitable: often the volume and lack of structure reflect inadequate attention to research design and focus at an early stage, resulting from qualitative researchers' tendency to overemphasize discovery at the expense of cumulative knowledge building, which we criticized in Chapter 2. The situation has not been helped by the slow development of methodological literature, as we noted in Chapter 4. As a result, a large element of trust has frequently been called for in evaluating the analytic work that has been done in producing a final report:

> The full weight of evidence for a given conclusion is not usually presented. The observer's conclusions often have a *prima facie* validity, a "ring of truth" but the reader of his research report has no way of knowing whether a solid basis of fact underlies this. The reader does not have the data available with which to convince himself and must rely on his faith in the researcher's honesty and intelligence. (Becker and Geer 1960:270)

The practice of analysis involves searching for ways to reduce the "full weight of evidence" to manageable proportions for a final report and to demonstrate the researcher's credibility to the reader.

THE "FULL WEIGHT OF EVIDENCE"

Quantitative studies typically solve the question of data reduction through tabulation or the use of summary measures. It is not necessary to read every single questionnaire or attitude inventory because their content can be summarized as a series of statistics. In principle, every single piece of data contributes directly to the findings through its contribution to these summary numbers.[1] There is no direct equivalent in qualitative studies, although simple tabulations are sometimes used to explore particularly well-marked phenomena [e.g., Silverman (2000:145–47) on the relative length of consultations in private cancer clinics compared with those run by the U.K. National Health Service]. The data extracts reproduced in reports have to "stand for" the population of available data, much as a sample survey "stands for" the population that it purports to represent.

Nevertheless, there are strong similarities in the processes of quantitative and qualitative analysis (Cicourel 1964). Both begin by classifying or categorizing their raw data. There is a real difference here in that quantitative researchers will normally have deductively specified the categories in advance. It is sometimes said that a good quantitative study design has all the final tabulations defined within in it, leaving only the actual numbers to be filled in once the data are available. Qualitative researchers have traditionally tended to induce the categories they use after their data have been collected, if not necessarily at the very end of a study then at least subsequent to notes or recordings being made. Quantitative researchers present their summaries of the contents of these classes numerically, while qualitative researchers present their findings through the selection of examples, which may be designed either to demonstrate the "typical" case or the range of variation. Both types of research then further summarize the results by respecifying them in theoretical terms so that the findings of one study can be generalized to a wider frame of reference. This frame can then be used deductively either to structure further research by proposing an initial set of classes or categories whose applicability can be tested under different environmental conditions, or to inform policy or practice as a basis for more or less robust predictions about the likely consequences of particular actions. Let us consider each of these stages—categorization, representation, and generalization—in turn.

WHERE DO CATEGORIES COME FROM?

Survey researchers usually invest a good deal of effort at the beginning of their study in developing the categories that they will subsequently use in analysis. These will be linked to previous studies, perhaps drawing from banks of questions or measurement scales that have been used previously in this or related fields. Where such resources are not available, researchers will consider what hypotheses arise from previous studies or from relevant theory and how these can be operationalized. In many classic accounts of qualitative research, such preparation is considered irrelevant, unnecessary, and positively inappropriate. The categories are said to emerge from within the data. Typically, researchers will begin by reading over the material they have collected to see what strikes them as particularly interesting. Having found one item, they will then look for others that may be similar or different. Similar cases will prompt questions about what properties they share. Different cases will prompt questions about what is present or absent that might contribute to the differences. Glaser and Strauss (1967:101–16) describe this as the constant comparative method, although it is basically a version of Mill's account of induction, described in Chapter 2. As the process unfolds, the cases are assembled into categories that share common features. The identification of these features may suggest an underlying structure of organizing principles that relates the categories to one another in systematic ways.

In such accounts of qualitative data analysis, the process by which "something particularly interesting" in the data is identified is rarely explicated. If we consider what is involved in seeing that something is "particularly interesting" though, it is clear that this process cannot be quite as naive as it is sometimes presented. One way of understanding this is by thinking about what is involved in seeing that things are not "particularly interesting," that they are unremarkable, unworthy of notice, and utterly mundane. In a lecture given in 1970, Sacks discusses what is involved in "being ordinary":

> In the first instance, there's an easy answer: Among the ways you go about doing "being an ordinary person" is spending your time in usual ways, having usual thoughts, having usual interests, etc.; so that all you have to do, to be an "ordinary person" in the evening, is turn on the TV set. It's not that it *happens* that you're doing what lots of ordinary people are doing, but that you know the way to do "having a usual evening" is to do that. It's not just that you're selecting "Gee, I'll watch TV tonight," but you're making a job of and finding an answer to, how to do "being ordinary tonight". ... We can see, then, that it's a job. You have to know what anybody/everybody is doing; doing ordinarily. And you have to have that available to do. ... So there's a business of being an "ordinary person," and that business includes attending the world, yourself, others, objects, so as to see how it is that it's a usual scene. (1995:ii, 216–18)

One of the things we learn as we grow up is how to fit actions to contexts in such a way as to avoid others thinking that our behavior is strange. Later in the lecture Sacks uses the example of deciding to study a wall in detail for the afternoon. If we are a prisoner in solitary confinement, then this may appear to be a reasonable thing to do. If we have taken LSD—remember the date of the lecture—it may seem odd but intelligible. If neither of these circumstances applies, then we might consider that this is indicative of some disordered relation to reality, behavior that we often describe as a symptom of mental illness. Behaving in a context-appropriate way is central to being ordinary or unremarkable.

Our knowledge of the relationship between actions and contexts cannot, of course, be perfect. We cannot know all the situations in which we will find ourselves in the future course of our lives. As children, growing up in particular times and particular environments, we learn some general strategies for being unremarkable. As we move into new environments, these strategies may be refined or modified: context-appropriate action in a hospital is not the same as context-appropriate action in one's own kitchen or bedroom. We also learn appropriate ways of dealing with novelty or uncertainty—this is the de facto solution to our imperfect knowledge of future contexts. Our knowledge of context-appropriate action is what allows us to identify context-inappropriate action, behavior that is, in this setting, strange, unusual, exotic, inexperienced, or otherwise remarkable and noticeable.

Sometimes the identification of context-inappropriate action parallels the work of participants in a setting. Light describes an incident during the induction of residents at a major U.S. university psychiatric center:

> Blumberg (the clinical director), a portly man with a soft voice, gently asked each resident to "introduce yourself and tell us a little about yourself."
>
> The first resident replied by giving his name, where he went to medical school, where he interned, and perhaps his interest in psychiatry. This cautious professional answer to so leading a question was picked up by each resident in turn. There is, of course, a rhythm to this process of introduction. About the fifteenth man had said who he was, where he went to school, that he interned at Children's Hospital, when Blumberg asked, "Do you like to play with children?"
>
> The resident who had stood up to take his turn, gaped, wordless, his eyes darting as if to find a quick escape. The tension of hushed silence mounted and then he replied, "Yes." As the embarrassed resident sat down, a few snickers came forth. Then a wave of laughter. The residents next to me looked quickly at each other; some whispered. Blumberg eased the moment with a joke and asked the next resident to introduce himself.
>
> During the rest of the day and the weeks to follow, a number of residents talked about this moment and puzzled. Was Blumberg making a psychiatric joke? Why put a resident on the spot? The victim thought Blumberg showed indiscretion. Later in the year, residents clearly knew what had happened: Blumberg had given a first, dramatic taste of psychoanalytic technique for exposing unconscious motives. What might have been taken as a quip in another setting was taken here to illustrate Blumberg's powers to disarm and to indicate that a psychiatrist's unconscious is a shared, professional concern. (1980:66–67)

This is quite a polished data extract: Light has clearly sought dramatic language to capture the drama of the moment. However, the core of it is a three-line exchange between the clinical director and a hapless resident:

Blumberg: Do you like to play with children?
(Pause of unknown duration)
Resident: Yes.

Although Light has not given us the details of the preceding talk, he describes it in a way that shows how Blumberg cuts into its established pattern with an utterance everyone marks as apparently inappropriate— first by the resident's silence, then by the laughter, and verbal and nonverbal interaction among his peers. These markers are Light's evidence that everybody in the context hears this utterance as significant. What, though, does it signify? The residents themselves debate this. Is there a double meaning here—"play" both in the sense of engage in innocent games and in the sense of sexual abuse? Why pick on this particular resident? In the course of the residency experience, both Light and the residents eventually come to see that this is a pedagogic technique. One of the issues that instructors confront residents with is the openness of their own behavior to the kind of diagnostic tools that they use on their patients. Blumberg's intervention both announces the way in which trainees will be required to examine themselves in the course of their residency and the potential for emotional distress that this will generate. To what extent are the residents' professed desires to "do good" merely covering up unconscious desires for power and self-gratification? Blumberg has interrupted an "ordinary" process of introductions, familiar to all of us with experience of new groups in organizational settings. The result makes his comment stand out both to the group and to the observer and leads both to seek to understand what this interruption might signify. That significance only unfolds, for both participants and observer, as the residency progresses and this event is set alongside later events as an instance of a pattern of behavior by supervising clinicians and faculty, which residents will, in their turn, come to use with patients.

Light started from behavior that was noticeable to participants as inappropriate. He developed his analysis from the evidence of their puzzlement at this breach of what, following Sacks's analysis that we cited earlier, we could call an "ordinary" way of doing things. However, an alternative strategy is to start from knowledge of previous research on comparable, or contrasting, settings and its formulations of context-appropriate behavior. Dingwall and Murray's (1983) discussion of categorization in emergency care, which was briefly introduced in Chapter 2, began in precisely this way. A previous study by Jeffery (1979) had proposed that "bad" patients—

"rubbish" as the staff called them—broke one or more of four rules: patients must not be responsible for their own condition; patients should be restricted in reasonable activities by the condition they complain about; patients should see illness as undesirable; patients should cooperate in treatment. Dingwall and Murray applied these rules to their data and discovered that they were consistently broken by one set of patients who did not then receive the kind of dismissive or even punitive treatment offered to "bad" patients in Jeffery's study. These patients were all "children"—the quotation marks emphasize that this was a social category, not a simple chronological one, as demonstrated by our later discussion of a child thought to be malingering. As a result, Dingwall and Murray revised and elaborated Jeffery's analysis. The noticeability to them of the category "children," and their exemption from the rules that would otherwise apply, depended upon their prior knowledge of a widely cited previous study in another setting and of the categories of "ordinary behavior" that its author had formulated.

So far, we have discussed situations in which behavior was identified as remarkable by the participants in the setting or was seen as remarkable by the researcher, in the context of existing knowledge. Often, however, the analysis of behavior in context does not have such obvious starting points. In order to overcome this, the training of qualitative researchers is designed to establish a way of viewing action that is in some sense *orthogonal* to that of the people who are actually involved in the context being studied. Qualitative researchers try to make the familiar strange, to see their own society as if they were anthropologists studying a different society or as if they were Martian anthropologists trying to understand the people of Earth. It is only through this self-conscious distancing from the conventional assumptions of ordinary, everyday life that we can describe these and explore how they work. In scientific terms, the objective of much qualitative research is to define what people in particular contexts *know* to be appropriate action, how they *activate* this knowledge, and how this process results in *judgments* about what is normal or deviant, judgments that normally arise from *interaction* between judge and judged. So a qualitative researcher's first question when confronted with a piece of data is often, How do the actions represented by this data come to happen in the way that they do? rather than, What is happening? or Why is it happening? We shall look at some examples of this process in more detail later in this chapter.

DO CAQDAS PACKAGES HELP?

Many claims have been made in recent years for the potential value of computer-assisted qualitative data analysis software (CAQDAS) in supporting this process of categorization. As a tool, the computer has a longer history in qualitative data analysis than many current users realize. For example, Dingwall used simple indexing programs on mainframes for his doctoral dissertation in the early 1970s and for his study of agency decision-making in child protection during the early 1980s. These programs automated the traditional methods of cut and paste or Cope Chat™ cards. In the early days, qualitative researchers would transcribe their fieldnotes using multiple carbon copies on a typewriter so that some could be cut up and physically shuffled into piles representing categories of observation. For a short time, there was some experimentation with pasting notes onto proprietary (Cope Chat™) cards punched around the edge with holes. A category would be assigned to each hole, which would then be clipped out with a special tool. Rods like knitting needles, were then passed through these holes and the pack shaken so that, where holes had been clipped out, relevant data would literally fall from the stack. Dingwall's projects gave each page of the transcribed fieldnotes a unique reference code and listed topics that occurred there: the software simply generated an index of locations at which material on specified topics was to be found. Since that time there has been considerable development of packages like NUD*IST™, ETHNOGRAPH™, HYPERRESEARCH™, ATLAS/ti™, and QUALPRO™. Although these vary in detail, they now allow text to be loaded and manipulated electronically, so that materials can be coded and retrieved on-screen. Some can also handle sound and video files. These packages also support Boolean searches and visualizations of code structures, which can be the basis of either combination or disaggregation of categories. (Useful information on the current state of the market can be found at http://caqdas.soc.surrey.ac.uk/index.htm.)

Two different claims are made about the benefits of CAQDAS packages. One is a simple matter of efficiency, that they allow data to be manipulated more quickly than traditional methods. This is probably true, at least for large datasets, although our experience, and that of our graduate students, is that the efficiency gains need to be set against the time required to learn the package, format the data, and enter the codes (see also Kelle & Laurie 1995). Electronic handling may also offer some security against data loss. Some possible topics of analysis were deliberately abandoned in Dingwall's child abuse project because of a lack of confidence that twelve hundred sheets of paper could be pulled out of a set of about seven thousand and then successfully replaced in order to look at the next topic. This does not happen with modern software, although disk back-up is obviously vital. However, there is also a good argument that some data-sets may not be large enough to justify the labor involved in coding them. Many qualitative Ph.D. theses are based on thirty to fifty interviews plus various documents and possibly a small amount of observational data. It is questionable whether CAQDAS packages offer any efficiency gains in such circumstances. A contemporary version of cut and paste using multiple photocopies and colored highlighters may be quite adequate for the task.

More controversially, some developers have claimed that CAQDAS fundamentally transforms the analytic process, particularly through its visualization capacities. This claim needs to be treated with some caution. At one level, it can seem like the common misapprehension among less-skilled quantitative researchers that running data through a package like SPSS™ constitutes doing analysis. SPSS™ is, of course, merely a tool whose value depends upon the skill with which it is used. The software is only as good as the questions that are asked of it and the judgment that is applied to its output. Software alone will not tell its user whether a particular cross-tabulation or regression is a sensible thing to do: it will simply carry out the programmed task. Similarly, it will not tell the user how to interpret results and what intellectual weight to attach to statistical levels of significance. The same is true of CAQDAS packages, as one or two of our graduate students have discovered to their chagrin. Loading and coding is only the first part of the task: interrogating and interpreting require as much investigator input as ever. A claim that a particular package was used may not, in itself, tell a reader or reviewer very much about the quality of the thought that has gone into a particular piece of work.

At another level, a reasonable claim can certainly be made that the requirements of loading and coding mean that a dataset has been read closely and that, to the extent that the coding has been done rigorously and meticulously, it has been exhaustively searched for all possible exemplars of a category. This may help to address the next issue that we deal with, namely, the representativeness of the data extracts selected for presentation. Any claim, though, that the visualization process has led to a qualitatively superior analysis is likely to be more contestable (Lonkila 1995). The patterns constructed by the analyst in linking codes, or by the software in listing co-occurrences of codes, are not necessarily intrinsic to the data (Seidel 1991:112). They are the product of the coding process and the coders' decisions about what may or may not be significant just as much as the official statistics that we discussed in Chapter 4. The use of CAQDAS packages may help to ensure that the "full weight of evidence" has been reviewed: it does not guarantee that the evidence relates to anything that is analytically important, nor that the analyst has avoided introducing patterns into the data to which the people whose behavior has been captured in the fieldnotes, documents, or interviews do not orient. In terms of our previous discussion, CAQDAS packages cannot tell us what is interesting in our data. At best, it can help us to mark things that we identify as interesting and to find them again easily.

WHAT ARE "REPRESENTATIVE DATA"?

One of the recurrent complaints of qualitative researchers is the lack of space offered by most book and journal publishers to present their data as fully as they would like. This is not as malign a process as some of the more paranoid imagine: it is partly a result of producing texts at a cost that the market can bear and partly the result of reader preferences. Ironically, of course, many of those who complain about space pressure are also the first to complain about prolixity in others' work when they come to read it! A one-to-one correspondence between data and published analysis is also somewhat at odds with the social scientist's mission to identify a smaller number of principles that generate the behavior recorded in the data. There are rare occasions, particularly in life-history studies, which we mentioned in Chapter 5, where such extensive reports may be justified, with commentary reserved for a separate chapter or section of a book. At its heart though, analysis is fundamentally about selection and reorganization.

Once it is accepted that it is normally impossible to include all the available and potentially relevant data collected in the course of a qualitative study, it is necessary to consider what principles of selection might be adopted. Three seem to be particularly important: including both exotic and mundane events; including events with sufficient context to allow alternative interpretations; including negative or deviant cases where these exist.

An important difference between journalism and qualitative research is the priority that the latter gives to the routine and everyday over the exotic. As we saw in Chapter 4, for example, the work of Bosk (1979) and Millman (1976) on institutional responses to medical errors was not intended to expose malpractice in particular cases so much as to use the anonymous study of individual events to understand why it can be difficult for surgical teams and hospitals to learn from them. There is always a temptation in qualitative research reports to choose the most exciting, dramatic, or morally outrageous example of some category rather than the most ordinary or mundane. It makes for a livelier account and greater reader engagement. Some of this is evident in the extract from Light's work quoted above. When he writes about "The resident who ... gaped, wordless, his eyes darting as if to find a quick escape," we are getting a dramatic rendition as much as a behaviorized description. However, Light is also showing how an exotic event can be used to make sense of everyday events. This is obviously a striking example of something that became part of the ordinary experience of the psychiatric residents. It stands out as their first encounter with a pedagogical trick that was routinely used by their instructors. As Light explains this, his analysis shifts from a possible expose of Dr. Blumberg as insensitive, overbearing, etc., to show how this event defines and characterizes a routine part of the residency experience. Toward the end of the book, he questions the implications more directly but only after he has explained how this style of teaching is embedded in the organization of the residency program. It is not an individual pathology of Dr. Blumberg but part of the institution's logic and, hence, not easily susceptible to reform in isolation from its context. More generally, however, a representative presentation of data will be dominated by data extracts that people in the setting being studied would consider entirely unremarkable.

Data extracts will also contain sufficient context to justify the interpretations applied to them and, ideally, to provide for the possibility of alternative readings, even if those readings are also discussed and discarded as we suggest below. If we look again at the extract from Light, we can see how the key exchange is embedded in a description of its context—the preceding pattern of introductions and the subsequent group reactions and analyses. It is only by showing this context that the apparent inappropriateness of Blumberg's question stands out—the fifteenth resident was not allowed to proceed in exactly the same manner as the fourteenth and the sixteenth. Light's description of the various interpretations offered by the other residents also suggests the possibility of alternative readings to the one that he proposes. The presentation here could have been improved by a reference forward in the book to other occasions when the same pedagogic trick was pulled, as evidence for the analysis preferred by the author, but the basis for his preference comes through with reasonable clarity. The precise form and nature of the contextual information that is included will vary somewhat with the nature of the data and the point being made. In an interview transcript, for example, it may be sufficient simply to include the question that an informant's response addresses rather than just presenting the answer on its own without knowing how it may have been shaped by the original question.

Finally, a representative presentation of evidence is likely to include consideration of negative or deviant cases. Are there occasions when the analysis being proposed does not fit the empirical data? What is peculiar about these cases? Can they be used to define limits on the generalizability of the central argument? Do they suggest some extra elements that need to be added to the analysis? Dingwall and Murray, for example, discuss the case of Francis, a thirteen-year-old boy who has presented at the emergency room on nine occasions in two years with trivial injuries and receives relatively punitive treatment by the staff instead of the general exemption from responsibility observed in relation to other children. The junior doctors (equivalent to interns in the United States) dealing with the case draw the researcher's attention to a communication from the boy's general practitioner who declares that he has told the boy and his mother that these injuries are normal for a child of his age and do not merit emergency attention. This frames his condition as one for which he can be held responsible and managed as if he were an adult presenting with a trivial injury. The authors also note the way in which a junior nurse is diverted from her initial assumption that the boy should be treated sympathetically as a child by a signal from the treating doctor. By exploring how this case comes not to fit the analysis that they are developing, Dingwall and Murray strengthen confidence in the analysis itself and in its limits of relevance. They also address the elements of credibility that we deal with later in this chapter.

WHAT DOES "THEORY" MEAN?

A great deal of theoretical writing in the social sciences and humanities takes the form of "Just-So" stories. The genre is named after the work of the English writer Rudyard Kipling, whose book *Just-So Stories* was first published in 1902. In it he offers fanciful accounts of how the leopard got his spots, how the camel got his hump, how the rhinoceros got his skin, and so on. One form of scholarly work involves trying to explain how we came to have the kind of society and institutions that we experience around us every day. How was "the modern world" created? What is the "transition to postmodernity" doing to that world? How does our experience of "risk society" affect our daily lives? Much of this writing has a highly normative character—usually of a rather pessimistic nature. Sociology, in particular, has a well-deserved reputation for being a remarkably glum discipline, well-equipped to see the faults in any society and reluctant to see any benefits. In the context of this book, however, we are using "theory" in a rather different sense. Specifically, we are using it more with the meaning of "empirical generalization" or, in a slightly more technical sense, "second-order account." What do we mean by this?

The primary data of qualitative research are, broadly speaking, first-order accounts. That is to say, they are direct descriptions or reproductions of some set of events by people who participated in them or observed them directly. As we explained in Chapter 4, in the strictest sense, only direct observations are first-order data with documents and interviews at some remove. However, we do not need to insist on this difference at this point: the crucial distinction is between descriptions of events that emphasize their unique and idiosyncratic nature and descriptions that show them to be instances of types or categories, where the central concern is with the categories themselves and their relations with each other. It is these categories and the relations between them that make up the basis of second-order accounts.

If we go back to the research on emergency rooms, for example, Jeffery begins his analysis by noticing the staff category of "rubbish," a type of patient that seems to be the same as "crocks" or "gomers" in U.S. studies

(Becker et al. 1961; Mizrahi 1986). He then asks what the varied individuals who are described in this way have in common and identifies the four rules that they break. In the process, "rubbish" ceases to be purely a category used by one set of emergency room staff in one U.K. hospital. "Rubbish" is now proposed as a generic name for a type of patient that has appeared in previous studies without being formally defined in this way and that may be expected to occur elsewhere, at least wherever these four rules are relevant. Dingwall and Murray take over this description, pointing to a number of logical and empirical difficulties, and construct a more elaborated version that links "rubbish" patients to "children" and to "good" patients, showing how the same rules can be developed to produce a logical set.

As both papers note, this process begins to suggest that "rubbish" patients have considerable similarities to "unpopular" patients as this category was being developed at about the same time (see Kelly & May 1982). There are also echoes of the more generic discussions of the "sick role" by Parsons (1951) and Goffman (1969), which try to define the conditions under which people may properly claim the support of others during a period of dependency. Although the precise linkages remain to be worked out in detail, the process of doing so would join some very precise observations of everyday behavior by health workers in a variety of settings to some rather general problems for anyone concerned with policy at the highest level, namely ensuring the equitable delivery of health services and defining the proper boundary of the social provision of health care. What is the point at which either a nationalized health service or an insurance-based system should cease to make provision for people who consider themselves to be in need but whose claims are questioned by others? How can this boundary be managed in a way that is politically and morally legitimate—something that, in the end, comes down to the way in which individual providers deal with individual patients presented to them? We shall look at another example of such linkage in the final section of this chapter.

The key point is that qualitative research rarely provides a definitive answer to policy or management questions so much as it improves the formulation of the questions and specifies the implications of possible answers. The management question, What do we do with "rubbish" patients? turns out to involve some rather hard thinking about what kind of service is being provided and why some people fall into this category. The responses may include a reformulation of the service and diversion of "rubbish patients" to a more appropriate intervention, attempts to reeducate the "rubbish" to change their consultation behavior and more or less coercively presented denials of service. Once a management decision is made, the existing body of research may be able to help with its implementation: what kinds of alternative interventions might be possible? What sorts of reeducation might be effective? How can service be denied without violent confrontations that threaten staff and other patients? Theory provides the way in which the specific experience of other sites can be transported to the one currently posing such questions.

THE "HONESTY OF THE RESEARCHER"

We have moved through some of the issues involved in data reduction, from the original corpus of fieldnotes, transcripts, or audio or video recordings to the formulation of empirically grounded generalizations that allow the experience of one or a small number of cases to be transferred to others as a point of departure for research, management, or other interventions. However, as Becker and Geer pointed out, this still leaves important questions of trust. How do readers and users of research reports know that this process has been carried out conscientiously and with integrity? We shall return to this question again in Chapter 9, when we discuss the evaluation of qualitative research reports. It will, though, repay some examination at this point. Let us return again to the passage from Light's research. What features would lead us to see this as honest recording and analysis?

Two features seem to be important: the precision of the language used to describe the event, the setting and the participants; and the transparency of the reasoning from data to conclusions.

Precise language may not absolutely distinguish the scientific description from a piece of realist fiction.

> "It isn't, it isn't cancer, is it, Doctor? I haven't got cancer?" Pavel Nikolayevich asked hopefully, lightly touching the malevolent tumour on the right side of his neck. It seemed to grow almost daily and yet the tight skin on the outside was as white and inoffensive as ever.
> "Good heavens no, of course not," Dr. Dontsova soothed him, for the tenth time, as she filled in the pages of his case history in her bold handwriting. Whenever she wrote, she put on her glasses with rectangular frames rounded at the edges, and she would whisk them off as soon as she had finished. She was no longer a young woman; her face looked pale and utterly tired. (Solzhenitsyn 1971:9)

This passage from the opening to Solzhenitsyn's great novel, *Cancer Ward*, which uses health care to explore the corruption of Soviet socialism, has something of the same exactitude as Light's description of the introductory meeting of the psychiatric residents. Solzhenitsyn invents a dialogue between Pavel Nikolayevich and Dr. Dontsova, which is rendered as precisely as the exchange between Dr. Blumberg and the unnamed resident.

The behavior of both actors is described meticulously—touching the tumor and writing the case history. We have a physical depiction of Dr. Dontsova, the business with her glasses and its implied link to her age and facial features. She is captured as a woman who would like to pass for younger, as one who does not need the glasses to compensate for aging eyesight, but whose countenance belies this. In the same way, Light immortalizes Dr. Blumberg as a "portly man with a soft voice."

Both authors draw a portrait in words: indeed, as we noted earlier, Light's language is, if anything, the more vivid. The crucial difference lies in the authors' claimed access to the mental states of the actors. Solzhenitsyn allows us to infer this in the case of Dr. Dontsova, from his description of her appearance and mannerism, but tells us what is in Pavel Nikolayevich's thoughts as he touches the tumor—growing daily without revealing its true malevolence to the outside observer. Light, however, does not presume to know what was in Dr. Blumberg's mind when he challenged the resident. Indeed, the problem of determining what his intervention might have meant becomes central to the analysis: it is a problem for residents and fieldworker alike.

The second feature of research reports that will strengthen our confidence in their integrity relates to the transparency of the reasoning involved in the analysis. In the extract from Light, we can notice his even-handedness. The victim thought that Blumberg had behaved badly but Light withholds judgment on this claim. He does not simply rush into a provictim, or proauthority, stance but expects to find a rationale for Blumberg's behavior. He lays out the range of interpretations that were current among the residents. Was this simply a joke? Did it have some purpose that was not apparent to them at the time? Eventually, Light notes that the residents come to a consensus that they have experienced a pedagogic technique, which he links to other, unspecified, observations to sustain the generalization that the program makes the unconscious of each resident into public business, at least for instructors and peers. This might have been even more persuasively presented by making clearer linkages to the data that sustained the final interpretation of Blumberg's intervention but such compression is often an inevitable part of the compromise between exhaustive presentation of material, the economics of publication and the attention span of readers—*Becoming Psychiatrists* runs over four hundred pages as it is!

While, in principle, fiction writers could both eschew claims to access mental state and make their reasoning transparent in the way that Light does, it is very difficult to do so consistently. A key trigger for the suspicion with which Castaneda's Ph.D. dissertation about sorcery in the American Southwest came to be treated was his apparent narrative omniscience and entry into the minds of his characters, notwithstanding his claims to have used magic and traditional psychotropics to achieve this experience (Castaneda 1970; De Mille 1976, 1980). This is not to say that one could not write a fiction that was purely exterior, although the very concept of the novel is normally thought to turn on the possibility of exploring the psychology of its characters by entering into the private processes of thought that are inaccessible in everyday interaction. With qualitative data, there should always be the ultimate safeguard of referring legitimate reviewers to the original fieldnotes or recordings and, except where there are overriding concerns for the safety or security of participants, recontacting the people whose actions are documented in them. As we shall see in Chapter 9, the latter is no guarantee that the scenes will be exactly as they recall but it is some form of insurance. Ironically, the greatest threat to the possibility of such checks on fraud or fabrication comes from the desire of ethical review boards to see original data destroyed as rapidly as possible. The conflict between research integrity regulations and human subjects protection is likely to be a point of some tension in coming years.

RECORDING AND RECENT DEVELOPMENTS
IN ANALYTIC PROCEDURES

The introduction of audio- and video-recording technologies to qualitative research since the 1960s has made possible a number of innovations in the process of analysis. As we promised in Chapter 4, this section will examine these innovations in some detail, partly to underline the extent to which qualitative work can, and has, moved away from some of the intuitive traditions that have been discussed earlier. In doing so, we shall also demonstrate how various kinds of interaction analysis get done.

Traditionally, researchers treated doctor-patient interaction as a site where doctors exercised power over patients. The earliest social scientific writing on this topic, by Talcott Parsons (1951), based on his observations of medical practice in the Boston area in the late 1930s and 1940s, emphasized the authority of the physician and his role as controller of access to the right to make dependency claims on other people. People had to defer to this gatekeeper in order to be defined as "sick" and entitled to claim special treatment from family, friends, or public assistance agencies. Later writers extended this into arguments that access to the "sick role" was actually regulated by physicians in the interests of capital (e.g., Waitzkin 1991) or patriarchy (e.g., Oakley 1980; Todd 1989; Fisher 1995). Part of the evidence for these claims has been derived from recordings of doctor-patient interaction. These are claimed to show a systematic pattern of asymmetry, in that doctors ask more questions than patients (West 1984b), interrupt patients more than the reverse (West 1984a, 1984b), decide which topics are relevant to the consultation (Davis 1988), and so on [see ten Have (1991) and Maynard (1991a, 1991b) for further examples]. This asymmetry is read off as indicative of the exercise of power and authority by the physician over the patient.

The following example of this kind of critical analysis is from Waitzkin (1991:77–79). The consultation appears to have been recorded sometime in the early 1980s. As background, it seems to be relevant to know that certain information is already shared between patient and doctor: the patient had a heart attack several months previously; he has since been convalescing on disability benefit; he has also been diagnosed as depressed; and his workplace union is coming to the end of its labor contract and threatening to strike over the renewal terms:

1. **Doctor:** How are things coming at work?
2. **Wife:** He hasn't been to work yet.
3. **Patient:** Well, you know, they prolonged it, they've extended the contract for ten days.
4. **Doctor:** Yeah.
5. **Patient:** Which is a good sign.
6. **Doctor:** Yeah.
7. **Patient:** From what I heard that's a good sign.
8. **Doctor:** So when would you be able to, when would they be ready to go if they approve a contract?
9. **Patient:** Oh, it'd probably be, well the contract runs out the 26th.
10. **Doctor:** Of this month, that's this Saturday.
11. **Patient:** That's this Saturday.
12. **Doctor:** And it's prolonged...
13. **Patient:** It'll be a week and a half.
14. **Doctor:** Yeah, so if they arrange something, they'll know by mid-June.
15. **Patient:** They should.
16. **Doctor:** Is that bugging you? The idea of going back to work?
17. **Patient:** Well ... actually I think I want to go back.
18. **Doctor:** Yeah, I think you should go back.
19. **Patient:** Actually, I think I want to go back, but then go back and go on strike? That seems to bother me.
20. **Doctor:** Yeah. But if you go back mid-June it won't, won't bother you.
21. **Patient:** No.
22. (Silence of unknown length)
23. **Doctor:** Just strip down to your waist, Mr. _____.

Waitzkin begins his analysis by noting that the doctor needs to be reminded that the patient has not returned to work after his heart attack (line 2). He argues that the doctor expropriates the patient's decision about returning to work (lines 18 and 20) and sustains this over a feeble reply, followed by a long pause (line 22) before the doctor begins a physical examination (not reproduced here). These conclusions are reached by a procedure that Waitzkin describes in the following way:

> Initially, each research assistant was to scan all the transcripts and to note those transcripts that dealt, even in minor ways, with the contextual issues of work; family life and gender roles; aging; sexuality, leisure, substance use, and other forms of pleasure seeking; and emotional problems. In this way, we hoped to accumulate transcripts illustrating the contextual issues of greatest interest. Within all transcripts, each research assistant also was to flag instances when either doctors or patients made statements that conveyed ideologic content or expressed messages of social control. (ibid.:68)

Like other critical authors, Waitzkin already knows what is of "greatest interest" and when statements convey "ideologic content" or express "social control." The recording simply makes possible a more accurate rendering of the original talk, which can then be inspected by his research assistants to locate instances of the events that he is interested in. There is no methodological innovation here. Waitzkin's work is located within the interpretive tradition of *verstehen* or role-taking introduced in Chapter 2, whose approach is based on an imaginative understanding of the actions being observed. This approach has had a very substantial influence on qualitative research. The observer asks him- or herself: "Suppose I were identically situated to the people I am observing, how would I understand their actions?" To be tendentious, we might say that the observer attempts to engage in an act of telepathy but is forced to settle for an approximation to it in the absence of a human faculty for this.

However, for at least two hundred years, social scientists have recognized that there is a possible alternative. The lack of a telepathic faculty is not just a problem for social scientists. It is a problem for everyone. As we have already noted, particularly in Chapter 2, when we interact with other human beings, we cannot possibly know exactly what is going on in their heads. How do we deal with this? We make inferences from their talk and behavior. Ordinarily we do this on the fly, so rapidly that it is a largely invisible process. Recording permits a different kind of analysis to be done that seeks to capture this process by repeated replaying of the sequences involved. While Waitzkin uses a recorder to produce a more literal record of a consultation than hand notes could achieve, he actually performs a relatively traditional kind of analysis. However, the same technology can be used to dig more deeply into the interaction itself.

By comparison with current standards, Waitzkin's notational conventions are rather limited so, although his transcript is easier to read, crucial information is lacking.[2] However, even on this version, it is possible to show an alternative reading that is never acknowledged. Has the doctor really forgotten that the patient is back at work? The timing of lines 2 and 3 is crucial to this. Are they actually alternative answers to the question in line 1? "How are things coming at work?" could be a reference either to the patient's experience of returning to his bench or to the progress of the labor negotiations. Notice the way in which it is actually the patient's answer that continues and structures the next part of the sequence.

Again, we do not quite know where the doctor's contributions at lines 4 and 6 are placed. The transcript makes them look like interruptions but they seem much more like "continuers," utterances that encourage a speaker to continue speaking on a topic. Syntactically, the patient's speech is continuous from lines 3 to 7 and the doctor only comes in with a new topic when the patient signals that he has finished by recycling line 5 as line 7. There are then several lines (8–15) where the patient and the doctor work out the timetable for a decision over the new labor contract. The patient has signaled optimism about a settlement and accepts (line 15) the doctor's summary of their exchange (line 14) as pointing to a mid-June date for knowing whether there will or will not be a strike. This is important because Waitzkin places a lot of weight on line 20 as the doctor asserting that a settlement will have been reached as a means of invalidating the patient's concern about going back to work. Line 20 is entirely consistent with the understanding reached between doctor and patient in lines 8–15. Waitzkin then reads line 16–21 as an assertion of labor discipline, of the doctor pressing the patient to return to work in the face of his uncertainty.

Even on this limited transcript, however, it should be noted that it is the patient who asserts a desire to return to work (line 17) in response to the doctor's question at line 16, which does not seem to presuppose any particular response. The doctor simply endorses the patient's choice. To the extent that the patient is "bothered," this seems to be more allied to discomfort with the idea of returning to work and then immediately coming out on strike. The significance of the silence at line 21 is simply not evident in the data. Waitzkin (ibid.:64–65) only has audiotape. The doctor may have been reading notes, preparing for the physical examination that follows this sequence, or checking test results. Certainly neither the doctor nor the patient treats the silence as significant in the next turn:

23. Doctor: Just strip down to your waist, Mr. _____.

Schegloff (1991, 1997)[3] lays out the more contemporary position that we have adopted in the analysis of these data. He contrasts the positions of those, like Waitzkin, who begin by stipulating the existence and relevance of power and status within and between social formations such as classes, ethnic groups, genders, age grades, and occupations and those who are trying to understand how participants are actually producing the observable social order through their moment-to-moment orientations to whatever matters are locally relevant at the time of production. The first of these

> allows students, investigators, or external observers to deploy the terms which preoccupy *them* in describing, explaining, critiquing, etc. the events and texts to which they turn their attention. There is no guaranteed place for the endogenous orientations of the participants in those events; there is no principled method for establishing those orientations; there is no commitment to be constrained by those orientations. However well-intentioned and well-disposed towards the participants—indeed, often enough the whole rationale of the critical stance is the championing of what are taken to be authentic, indigenous perspectives—there is a kind of theoretical imperialism involved here, a kind of hegemony of the intellectuals, of the literati, of the academics, of the critics whose theoretical apparatus gets to stipulate the terms by reference to which the world is be understood—when there has already *been* a set of terms by which the world was understood—by those endogenously involved in its very coming to pass. (Schegloff 1997:167)

Schegloff concludes with the stinging comparison of "critical" or "standpoint" analysis to those who speak of Columbus "discovering" America as if there were not indigenous people already there. In the same way, he implies sociologists are prone to "uncover" or "reveal" features in everyday life as if ordinary people were not already doing it quite adequately without any identifiable reference to these features. The task is not "to privilege sociology's concerns under the rubric 'social structure' but to discover them in the members' worlds, if they are indeed there" (1991:66).

The methodological innovation developed by Schegloff and others since the 1960s is founded on the recognition that, at its simplest, all face-to-face interaction rests on a three-turn structure and that modern recording technologies allow this to be captured in a way that was not previously possible. I say something; you respond to it; and I can then use the third turn to decide whether your response is adequate and adequately connected to what I said first. In that turn, I can either decide to move on or rework (repair) my first turn and hope you will respond more satisfactorily or ask you to explain (account for) your failure to link your turn in second position to my first utterance. This is a dynamic structure: the second turn for me is the first turn for you so that you can examine what I do in the third turn, from my position, as a second turn for you—and then use your next turn as a third position to comment on what I have done.

My sequence	=	Your sequence
1. My statement		
2. Your response	=	1. Your statement
3. My review	=	2. My response
		3. Your review

In reality, the process is often somewhat more complicated. Other parts can be inserted in the sequence and the third turn may be left empty if the speaker does not choose to use it. However, this description will serve as a starting point for showing how the problem of telepathy is solved.

Philosophers have long recognized that the meaning of an utterance is not determined by our intentions in producing it but by the way that it is understood by the people who hear it. Whatever I may have intended to say in the first position, I will only find out what hearers have decided that I said when I receive a response in the second position. That response, which the hearer assumes is appropriate and adequately connected to what I said, tells me how I have come across. If I intended something different, I can either try to say the same thing again, probably in a slightly different way, or I can ask the hearer to explain how he or she came to hear my first turn in a way that prompted him or her to respond in an unexpected fashion. The evidence for what each of us meant by what we said is not to be found in an imaginative reconstruction of what an observer thinks we might have meant but in the close study of the talk itself.

If we return to the reanalysis of Waitzkin's transcript, for example, we can see that the doctor's utterance in line 1 becomes a question not because of its grammatical form but because it elicits answers—competing second turns—in lines 2 and 3. Whether the doctor intended the meaning assumed by the patient is something that neither we nor the patient can ever know. However, we can see that the doctor uses the third position (line 4) to endorse the patient's response rather than the wife's and to encourage him to continue. The sequence through to line 7 makes line 1 into a question about the labor negotiations rather than a question about the patient's individual experience of work. When the topic changes, it is because the patient has reached what is a third position for him (line 7) and chooses not to pursue the topic further. The doctor's introduction of a new topic (line 8) does not cut the patient's talk off but responds to its abandonment. The same seems to happen at lines 15 and 16 and at line 21. The point is that, if there is an apparent asymmetry between doctor and patient, this seems to be as much the result of the patient deferring to the doctor as it is of the doctor cutting off the patient and imposing an agenda. The space for the doctor to change topics is collaboratively produced.

Examples of the examination of asymmetry in this alternative tradition can be found in work by Sharrock (1979), Heath (1992), and ten Have (1991). In this discussion, however, we want to focus on two further methodological points.

The first is the extent to which this approach does not preclude quite traditional forms of fieldwork. As we noted in Chapter 4, it is not possible to record everything everywhere. However, it is possible to transfer the findings and sensibility of interaction analysis to other kinds of data. The extract from Light's work earlier in this chapter is a good example. His fieldwork in the early 1970s stands on the cusp of these changes. At the core of the extract is a sequentially inappropriate utterance by Dr. Blumberg and the struggle to produce an appropriate next turn. It provides an introduction for both the author and the students to an environment where sequential coherence will frequently be in doubt, as a result of the challenging forms of interaction generated by psychotherapy, and where the recognition of competence will often turn on the ability to use psychotherapeutic theories to find coherence in apparently unconnected events, whether prompted by instructors or by patients.

The second, which is the obverse of the preceding comment, is that it does have quite serious implications for the analysis of interview data, as we noted in Chapter 5. Waitzkin's description of his analytic procedure takes an orthodox approach to qualitative interview data—cut the sections that deal with particular preselected topics, paste them together, and use the results to illustrate a narrative that is already decided upon. It is a curious qualitative perversion of the quantitative design that draws up all the tables in advance: the story is already written and the data are generated to fit. However, as we have shown, the production of talk in interaction and the determination of meaning are complex processes. Interviews are no different from any other form of face-to-face interaction (or mediated interaction if done by phone!). The talk that is captured on an audio or video recording is just as much a collaborative construction as the medical consultation taped by Waitzkin and reanalyzed in this chapter. As we stressed before, this does not mean that interview data are unusable: it does mean that they need to be used with great care and scrupulous attention to the extent to which the interviewer has prompted the data that he or she claims later to have discovered. The analysis of interview data must also be informed by the sensibility of interaction analysis.

CONCLUSION

We have reviewed key issues in the analysis of qualitative research data, and begun to consider the issue of how one might tell whether this had been done well or badly. The evaluation of qualitative research reports will be the core of Chapter 9. Before reaching this, however, it is also important to acknowledge that technical competence alone is not sufficient. As we have shown, in discussing the credibility of the researcher, good work is also in part an ethical commitment. Qualitative methods are often thought to present special ethical problems that restrict their employment in an increasingly regulated research environment. While we shall argue that some of this concern is misplaced, reflecting the limited understanding of both regulators and regulated of the imperatives of their own environment, it is undeniable that qualitative work does require a particular kind of ethical sensibility. The next chapter, then, will explore the ethical issues arising around contemporary qualitative research.

NOTES

1. In practice, of course, individual pieces of data are often excluded as "outliers," "missing values," "incomplete," etc.

2. Most comparable work now uses the system developed by Gail Jefferson, which is described in Jefferson (1984).

3. See also the exchange between Billig and Schegloff (1999), which continues the debate.

8

The Ethics of Qualitative Research

All research involving human participants raises ethical questions. What can researchers legitimately do to other human beings, whether in order to further knowledge or their own careers? What obligations do researchers have to those who take part in their research? What rights do research participants have? Are risks, however, minimal, ever justified? When the research relates to health, disease, and health care, these questions have particular force. In this chapter we shall examine the distinctive ways in which they apply to the practice of qualitative health research.

The relevance of these ethical concerns to researchers and the health professionals who can facilitate or withhold access to clients and/or settings is self-evident, but research commissioners may ask why they need to know about research ethics. It is a reasonable question. If commissioners are paying for specific information to be obtained by the use of a particular method, then they may simply take the view that research ethics are not really their concern. Indeed, if researchers raise ethical issues, commissioners may conclude that they are being overscrupulous and allowing personal values to get in the way of an ordinary commercial relationship. Researchers' reservations about what they are being asked to do may be dismissed as an excess of political correctness and mean that, mentally or literally, they are crossed off the list of people with whom commissioners are willing to do business in the future. Taking this line, however, opens research commissioners to significant political and legal risks and probably means that they will not be able to commission research from skilled and reputable investigators.

By "political risks" we do not exclusively mean direct intervention by government in commissioning activities, although this may well be the result. We are thinking more of the public image of the organization. Does it inspire confidence in its users and clients? Is it seen as a good place to work by the best-qualified professionals? Are social activists, interest groups or lobbyists provoked to target the organization's activities as examples of irresponsible behavior?

Ethical concerns have particular significance for both commissioners and practitioners of health research. People feel vulnerable when they are dealing with matters that concern their health. They share a lot of information about themselves with health care providers, information that they might prefer to keep private. If their condition is stigmatized, a breach of privacy may have seriously damaging consequences for their personal lives, employability, or access to personal finance and insurance products. Health care providers must show that they can be trusted with this information. Sick people also have to be able to trust the goodwill of the people or organizations who are involved in their care, whether directly as a doctor or nurse, or indirectly, as a manager or a supplier of drugs, devices, or other therapeutic materials. Research raises issues about the privacy of the information that people have shared with their care provider and about the good intentions of those involved in care. Do they really have the patient's welfare at heart or are they just concerned with their own professional or financial interests? An apparent indifference to research ethics may compromise patient trust in the integrity of an organization, a profession, or a particular individual care provider. Lack of trust can have real social and economic consequences if people desert your business or service for competitors who are seen to have more integrity, or if those people demand greater regulation of your activities.

There has been a striking growth of regulation governing research on humans in many developed countries since World War II. The United States has a particularly elaborate system. This has significant implications for both practitioners and commissioners of research. Although penalties for breaches of regulations tend to fall primarily on researchers, failure to ensure compliance with relevant regulatory standards may increase a commissioner's vulnerability to legal actions by people who believe that they have been harmed by research. Large payments in damages are real losses, compounded by the reputational harm that may arise from reports of the judgment or settlement.

Qualitative research is frequently thought to raise difficult ethical problems. In fact, it is not so much that the ethical problems are particularly difficult, or even specific to qualitative methods, as that regulatory systems have difficulty in dealing with the nature of the work. Quantitative researchers typically do more of their design up front, and can submit much more specific and detailed instruments and protocols for approval. Survey work, for example, is highly bureaucratized and able to incorporate regulatory controls into its internal management processes, although any experienced survey researcher will have a fund of stories about the difficulty of getting interviewers to stick to protocols! Qualitative research, particularly that using observational methods, is less suited to anticipatory regulation and depends much more on the situational ethical judgments of the investigator.

As a result, researcher training usually tends to have a more substantial ethical component so that people in the field are equipped to reason for themselves to an appropriate conclusion when presented with an ethical challenge. However, this can be difficult for regulators to accept. Ethical regulation has grown partly because of a decline in the public trust afforded to researchers. Qualitative researchers ask regulators to trust them to do the right thing. Regulators ask why they should. How can they distinguish between ethical and unethical research in using methods that are inevitably less precisely defined in advance?

This chapter begins by examining the U.S. regulatory system, which has a good deal in common with those operating in other countries. We try to understand why this system takes the shape that it does. We then examine some of the conflicts that have arisen between regulators and qualitative researchers and their relationship to ethical debates within qualitative research. Are different goals being pursued? Can qualitative methods be specified in ways that meet regulatory concerns without compromising their distinctive contribution?

A BRIEF HISTORY OF ETHICAL REGULATION

Contemporary ethical regulation originates in public reaction to the medical experiments conducted by German doctors during World War II and exposed by the Nuremberg Medical Trial of 1946–47. These experiments included injecting prisoners with deadly viruses, immersing them in freezing water, and forcing them to ingest poisons (Lifton 1986). Twenty-three physicians and medical administrators, many of them leading members of the German medical profession, were charged by the Allies with crimes against humanity (Annas & Grodin 1992:70–86). The doctors' defense focused on the lack of any generally accepted standards governing experimentation on human subjects. Their studies were, they argued, medically justified. The U.S. history, of forcible eugenic interventions and of experiments, relating to cholera, pellagra, and malaria, conducted on imprisoned criminals without voluntary consent, showed that there was little difference between the defendants' behavior and the way Americans had used captive populations as research subjects.[1]

Prosecution witnesses argued that commonly held ethical standards could be formulated, at least implicitly, and used to judge the defendants' actions (ibid.:102–3, 132–37). The weakness of their position, however, is illustrated in the minutes of a prosecution team meeting in July 1946. The

Allied prosecutors and their scientific witnesses found they needed to for-mulate "some broad principles ... for the use of humans as subjects in ex-perimental work" in order to prevent the trial from stirring "public opinion against the use of humans in any experimental manner whatsoever that a hindrance will thereby relate in the progress of science." Although the prosecution referred to guidelines published by the American Medical Association, these did not actually appear until nineteen days after the trial started and seem to have been inspired by witnesses preparing for the trial (Hazelgrove 2002).

Within its guilty verdict, the tribunal included a section, entitled "Per-missible Medical Experiments," which became known as the Nuremberg Code. In effect, this set out the principles that the prosecution had been forced to treat as largely tacit. It has been an important reference point for all subsequent attempts to establish an ethical basis for research on human subjects. Ten principles had to be observed if such research were to be morally, ethically, and legally justifiable. In particular, participation in re-search must be voluntary and based on adequate knowledge and under-standing of its nature, duration, purpose, methods, and potential hazards. Other principles stipulated that research must avoid all unnecessary physi-cal and mental suffering and that the degree of risk must always be pro-portionate to the humanitarian importance of the problem under study.

The actual impact of the Nuremberg principles during the immediate postwar years seems to have been limited. Some critics have gone so far as to argue that the Allies simply assumed that the Code did not really apply to them (Hazelgrove 2002). By the end of the 1950s, there was growing unease among sections of the medical and scientific communities. Harvard professor Henry Beecher attacked the ethical standards of clinical research in leading U.S. institutions through two widely read papers in 1959 and 1966 (Beecher 1959, 1966; see also Rothman 1993). These concerns were reinforced as other questionable studies came to light during the late 1960s and early 1970s. Three became particularly notorious: the Tuskegee Syphilis Study (Jones 1981); the Jewish Chronic Disease Study (Rothman 1993); and the Willowbrook State School Study (Rothman 1993). In all three studies, groups of particularly vulnerable patients had been subjected to potentially harmful treatments, without obtaining fully informed consent.

The National Institutes of Health (NIH) first published a statement of Policies for the Protection of Human Subjects in 1966, which introduced Institutional Review Boards (IRBs), whose role will be examined shortly. These policies were given regulatory force by the Department of Health, Education and Welfare (DHEW) in May 1974, just as Congress was pass-ing the National Research Act, which established the National Commission for the Protection of Human Subjects of Biomedical and Behavioral Re-search. This commission was charged to establish the ethical principles that should guide all research that involved human participants. In 1979, the commission published the *Belmont Report: Ethical Principles and Guidelines for the Protection of Human Subjects of Research*. The commissioners identified three core principles—beneficence, respect for persons, and justice—which are discussed below. In response to this report, the Department of Health and Human Services (DHHS, successor to DHEW) undertook a significant revision of the 1974 regulations. These were codified as Title 45, Part 46, of the Code of Federal Regulations in January 1981 and were further revised in 1983, 1991, and 2001. The 1991 revision created what is known as the Common Rule, a uniform code of research ethics regulations covering all federal departments and agencies.[2] Although this is strictly only applicable to federally funded or supported studies, it specifies that such work may only take place in institutions that show general compliance with the principles underlying the Common Rule in all their research and implement these through IRB review [Health Research Extension Act 1985 sec.491(a); 45 CFR 46.103(b)].

In practice, then, the United States has created a federal regulatory system, administered through a network of highly localized IRBs, that seeks to apply the principles spelt out in the Belmont Report to all biomedical or behavioral research involving human subjects. Qualitative researchers have frequently felt that the IRB system discriminates against them. We are skeptical about this claim, arguing that the problems lie more with IRB memberships than with the system itself. However, this may indicate a particular need for commissioners and consumers of qualitative health research to give explicit support to researchers working for them, including being prepared to press for the appointment of better-informed members to IRBs.

INSTITUTIONAL REVIEW BOARDS

Many qualitative researchers complain about what they see as IRBs' unhelpful attitude toward their work, and there is sufficient evidence to suggest that these grievances have a real foundation.[3] IRB obstruction could be a major barrier to the wider use of qualitative methods in health-related research. If these methods are to make the contribution that we advocate, it will be necessary to find ways of reconciling qualitative researchers and IRBs.

Every institution that conducts research and receives, or hopes to receive, federal funds must have an IRB whose composition and procedures have been approved by the federal department or agency funding the work or by the Office for Protection from Research Risks in DHHS on behalf of the federal government as a whole (45 CFR 46.103). Every IRB must have at least five members "with varying backgrounds to promote complete and adequate review of research activities commonly conducted by the institution." Membership should reflect diversity of race, gender, cultural, and professional backgrounds, and should include at least one person not affiliated with the institution [45 CFR 46.107–8]. The IRB is required to ensure that research minimizes risks to subjects, that risks are proportionate to benefits, that the selection of subjects is equitable, that informed consent is obtained and documented, and that there are adequate provisions for ensuring participants' safety, privacy, and confidentiality (45 CFR 46.111). IRBs are allowed a measure of flexibility in dealing with research that presents minimal risks and some discretion in the application of the provisions on informed consent (45 CFR 46.110, 116–17).

Timmermans's (1995) account of his experiences is typical of the complaints made by qualitative researchers. He sees himself as the victim of both the sort of methodological prejudices that we discussed in earlier chapters and the manipulation of the IRB to protect vested interests. As he notes, there is an alternative history of IRBs, which argues that they have more to do with protecting disciplinary boundaries, intra- and interprofessional hierarchies, and the public image of institutions than they do with the protection of human subjects (see also Mitchell 1993). Timmermans's goal was to carry out an observational study of resuscitative efforts in emergency departments as the basis of his doctoral dissertation (see Timmermans 1999). The project had already been approved by his university's IRB and by the IRB of one hospital, but he needed a second site and therefore applied to the IRB at a second hospital. Approval was given initially, but when Timmermans submitted a report and draft paper at his first six-monthly review, the IRB responded by suspending his authorization on grounds of concern over research quality, validity, maintenance of confidentiality, and institutional rights.

The issues of participant confidentiality had been triggered by a misunderstanding[4] and were quickly resolved, leaving the main conflicts over methodology and the public image of the hospital. IRB members were concerned that the study design had not taken an experimental form and that there were no statistical expressions of Timmermans's generalizations. They were also unhappy about Timmermans's portrayal of the contingency of ER work and the way in which this undercut the institution's preferred self- and public image of rational, protocol-driven scientific practice. Timmermans clearly had difficulty in responding to the first issue as a result of his position on the nature of truth and his identification with the relativist position that we have previously criticized. If all qualitative researchers can do is tell one more story about the world, then IRB members might be excused for wondering what the point is and what disciplines that story. The contingent nature of ER work is no surprise to anyone who has worked in such settings but there is no means of justifying a contested account of this from a relativist perspective. It is just my story versus yours. Nevertheless, Timmermans's experiences exemplify qualitative researchers' questions about the boundaries of IRB jurisdiction and the uses to which it is put.

However, it is far from clear that this is a problem with the system so much as with its execution. The *Institutional Review Board Guidebook* (Penslar & Porter 1993), which is the official manual for IRB members, has an extensive discussion of issues in the approval of behavioral and social research. Mostly, such research involves no physical risk, although there may be risks of social harm (damage to reputation) or psychological harm (damage from deception or disturbing information). There may also be some invasion of privacy. These issues are discussed in more depth below. Nevertheless, the *Guidebook* asserts, deception or invasion of privacy may be the only way in which research can be undertaken and must be considered potentially justifiable. Similarly, IRBs should avoid disapproving research simply because of its subject matter: their concern is with research methods and the protection of human subjects. A proposal to study unlawful or unethical behavior is not in itself problematic. The IRB may need to give particular attention to the protection of participants, but it may also need to use its discretion in relation to informed-consent requirements. While informed consent is, properly, the norm under the Common Rule, IRBs do have wide discretion to waive this where research would otherwise be impossible [45 CFR 46.116(c)2, 117(c)]. There is a particularly strong statement about fieldwork, quoted here in full:

> Fieldwork, or ethnographic research, involves observation of and interaction with the persons or group being studied in the group's own environment, often for long periods of time. Since fieldwork is a research process that gains shape and substance as the study progresses, it is difficult, if not impossible, to specify detailed contents and objectives in a protocol.
>
> After gaining access to the fieldwork setting, the ongoing demands of scientifically and morally sound research involve gaining the trust and approval of the persons being studied. These processes, as well as the research itself, involve complex, continuing interactions between researcher and hosts that cannot be reduced to an informed consent form. Thus, while the idea of consent is not inapplicable in fieldwork, IRBs and researchers need to adapt prevailing notions of acceptable protocols and consent procedures to the reality of fieldwork. IRBs should keep in mind the possibility of granting a waiver of informed consent.

While this does not *oblige* IRBs to adopt more flexible approaches, it certainly provides plenty of authority for them to do so. To the extent that qualitative researchers do encounter problems, these are more likely to reflect the difficulties, in smaller communities or institutions, of recruiting sufficiently knowledgeable IRB members or of ensuring an adequate level of training to familiarize them with the full range of their powers and duties. These are matters over which research commissioners and consumers are likely to have some influence.

RESEARCH ETHICS IN QUALITATIVE RESEARCH

If qualitative researchers are to earn the trust implied by the waiver of Common Rule requirements, it is essential that they demonstrate their adherence to the underlying principles of good practice, particularly those set out in the *Belmont Report*. Indeed, the case for a waiver will probably rest on a discussion in the proposal submitted to an IRB of the alternative methods that will be adopted to comply with these principles in the project that is being put forward. The case is unlikely to be met by the formulation of some alternative set of rules. The problems of a rule-governed approach have been extensively discussed (Barnes 1979; Cassell 1978 1979, 1982; Dingwall 1980; Finch 1986; House 1990; Punch 1994). The authors of the *Belmont Report* were sensitive to these and their focus on principles was intended to allow flexibility of interpretation in relation to specific projects. As they remarked:

> Rules are often inadequate to cover complex situations; at times they come into conflict, and they are frequently difficult to interpret or apply. Broader ethical principles will provide a basis on which specific rules may be formulated, criticized or interpreted.

The Belmont Report's principles are equally relevant to both qualitative and quantitative research in health, and have also served as the foundation of the "principlist" movement in the ethics of clinical practice, which is not discussed here (see Beauchamp & Childress 2001). There is no serious argument that these principles should not apply to qualitative studies, or that they cannot be applied, although it is important to recognize their cultural specificity.[5] The principles lay three clear duties on researchers:

Beneficence. Researchers have an obligation to ensure the well-being of research participants. They must maximize the possible benefits of research and minimize possible harms.

Respect for persons. People must be treated as autonomous agents able to make their own decisions about participation in research. Those whose autonomy is diminished in some way (because of age, illness, mental disability, or circumstances, such as imprisonment, that restrict their liberty) must be given special protection. The requirement that people should give

voluntary informed consent to research participation is a key expression
of this principle.

Justice. Researchers have a dual responsibility to research participants.
On the one hand, they must ensure that the potential benefits of research
are not distributed unfairly. On the other, they must avoid concentrating
the burdens and potential risks associated with research participation in
particular subgroups. The latter point reflects concerns about the exploitation of disadvantaged groups as subjects of research from which they were
less likely to benefit than members of more advantaged groups.

How can we understand each of these in relation to qualitative research?
What sorts of case might be made to an IRB?

Beneficence

This principle is concerned with the consequences of research. A study is
ethical if participants are not harmed by it, or if any harm they suffer is
outweighed by the benefits arising from the outcome. The researcher's
responsibility is to anticipate and avoid risks to participants while, at the
same time, ensuring the greatest possible benefit. In biomedical research
these principles are often translated into formal risk-benefit analyses: researchers are only allowed to proceed where they can clearly demonstrate
that the anticipated benefits of their work outweigh any possible risks.

Biomedical experimentation is well suited to formal risk-benefit analyses for a number of reasons. First, it is central to the logic of experiments
that the intervention is clearly specified in advance. This makes the precise
assessment of risk feasible. Second, the harm associated with trialing a new
drug or surgical technique is potentially very serious and, in some cases,
life-threatening. Third, any harm arising from biomedical experiments is
likely to be direct. It will be the consequence of the researcher's intervention in administering a drug or other treatment. In some cases, of course,
the consequences will take time to emerge so that the harm only becomes
obvious much later. Nevertheless the harm will be the direct effect of the
experimental manipulation and its relationship to the intervention can
normally be clearly specified.

Qualitative research differs on all three counts. As we have seen, its
approach to design is characteristically flexible and emergent. Within both
observational and interview studies, the researcher remains open to following up new leads and adjusting the research strategy accordingly. As in
experimental research, the qualitative researcher may intervene but that
intervention is marked by a much higher degree of indeterminacy. While
researchers may be expected to make general assessments of the potential

risk to participants at the outset of the study, this indeterminacy means that they must continually remake such assessments throughout the research. Changes in the research context, whether local or higher-level, may introduce new risks or reduce old ones. Changes in the focus of the research may threaten participants' well-being in ways that could not be anticipated at the outset of the study. Ethical decision-making in qualitative research is an ongoing activity and cannot be confined to an initial design stage.

While the risks associated with qualitative research are rarely of the same order as those associated with biomedical interventions, this does not mean that they are negligible. Indeed, as the *IRB Guidebook* notes, qualitative research introduces an additional range of possibilities for causing harm to participants. This social or psychological harm may, in some cases, be the direct result of the research activities. For example, interviews dealing with personal, sensitive, or stigmatized material may cause distress or embarrassment to informants. In a study of the effect on families of having a disabled child, Margaret Voysey (1975) interviewed the parents of twenty-two children with "relatively serious" and "probably permanent" physical and mental disabilities, on a number of occasions, over a period of approximately one year. The interviews covered topics such as the onset or diagnosis of the child's disability, encounters with medical agencies, and the impact of the disability on family life and encounters with others. Voysey reports that parents often became distressed during these interviews. It is fair to assume that the distress was provoked by the topics rather than by interviewer insensitivity. The material was, by its very nature, likely to be upsetting.

One could argue, although Voysey does not, that giving parents the opportunity to talk about these things was potentially therapeutic. Claims about the cathartic effects of research interactions should be treated with some caution (see, for example, Bar-On 1996). While some may welcome a sympathetic listener, others may experience more negative consequences. In most cases, the researcher will not be a trained counselor or therapist and may not have the skills to cope if the informant becomes seriously distressed. Even if he or she does have such skills, their use in this context raises concerns about blurring the relationship between research and therapy (Josselson 1996). Strategies can be adopted to minimize such risks: Bar-On (1996) describes how, in advance of interviews with the children of Nazi perpetrators, he identified local therapists to whom he could refer any informants who broke down during the interviews. Domestic violence researchers have long taken responsibility for identifying potential sources of support for research participants. This practice could usefully be extended to health research: the answer to IRB concerns about potential distress may not be to drop areas of questioning but to ensure that help is available to those who become distressed.

Sometimes, though, the risk of causing distress is too great to be justified. Renee Anspach's observational study of life-and-death decisions in the intensive care nurseries in two U.S. hospitals, which was referred to in Chapter 6 (Anspach 1993), is a case in point. Ideally, she would have interviewed the parents of all children about whom such decisions were being made. In the event, she interviewed far less than the optimal number of parents. For various reasons, many parents visited the nursery only infrequently. When they did, it was often in response to an invitation to attend a conference because a life-and-death decision was being made about their baby. On many occasions parents left the nursery in tears after their babies had died. Anspach decided that it was inappropriate to approach parents for interviews when they were crying or visibly extremely upset. This decision represented her attempt to "strike a balance between considerations of 'science,' on the one hand, and ethical and 'human' contingencies on the other" (ibid.:194). However, it was a matter for situational judgment rather than a research protocol.

Interviews may also be occasions when informants reflect on aspects of their situations to which they have not previously given much attention. In the process, they can come to reinterpret their experiences and relationships. Through interviews about their experiences of childbirth, for example, women may be led to question the interventions adopted by their medical attendants. They may redefine their obstetrician's behavior as overbearing or be provoked to resent their own lack of involvement in decision-making around their own or their babies' care. Whether one sees this outcome as a harm or a benefit depends upon one's point of view. It could be argued that the interview has eroded the trust between a woman and her obstetrician, which may have negative long-term consequences for her well-being. Equally, the outcome could be seen as beneficial insofar as it increases the woman's self-awareness. However, as Patai (1991) argues, any defense of research as "consciousness-raising" invites a charge of arrogance. What is the researcher's standing to declare that the preinterview state was one of lower consciousness, particularly given the uncertain relationship between interviews and the events they describe? Was the obstetrician really officious or has the woman been constrained by the interviewer to give an account that represents the obstetrician as officious in order to present herself as a rational informant?[6] Such claims may warrant particular attention from IRBs.

Anspach's (1993) study points to other possible harms. Her objectives included: identifying the major criteria that parents and professionals used in making decisions, examining the decision-making process, and exploring the impact of the hospital context, and the broader social and historical environment, upon these decisions. The first two objectives called for close observation of decision-making in practice and took Anspach into the "high-intensity" nursery, where children were critically ill. She reports her concern that she was "getting in the way" by asking nurses about particular babies when such distractions might have "potentially disastrous consequences" for children whose lives depended upon the activities in which the nurses were engaged. Anspach's response was to restrict her interactions with the nurses to other rooms where the babies were less critically ill and to the areas in which staff were taking their breaks and eating their meals.

Harm may occur as much as a result of what researchers fail to do as from what they actually do. Again, Anspach offers a useful example. For methodological reasons, her preferred role was that of a passive observer. However, she became aware that this passivity sometimes raised ethical problems. Evading a question or withholding information could harm (or at least fail to help) research participants. The situation was further complicated by the recognition that she was in danger of being cast in an expert role for which she possessed no particular competence or training. Anspach describes the rule of thumb she developed:

> To avoid actions that I thought would intervene in a decision *unless* I felt that my failure to intervene would be very damaging to research subjects or unless I had observed an event that I simply could not countenance. (ibid.:210, emphasis in original)

For the most part, this policy allowed her to adopt a passive role. However, there was at least one incident in which she felt obliged to be more active. She had interviewed both parents of a grossly malformed baby who had been in the nursery for several months without any apparent progress. She discovered that, contrary to their social worker's belief, both parents were pessimistic about the baby's future and worried about the baby's possible impact on their other six children. Anspach was concerned by the parents' distress and by the fact that the social worker appeared to be operating on the basis of misinformation. With the parents' permission, she encouraged the social worker to talk to them further. However, this did not produce any change in the management of the baby. In Anspach's own words, "The family's situation continued to plague me for several weeks" (ibid.). She then decided to intervene more actively:

> One day after rounds I approached the resident, who was taking care of Ramon, and said, "I'd like to ask you a question. What is the plan on the Martinez baby?" At that moment, I knew exactly what I was doing; I was aware that there was no plan and that my question might lead the resident to formulate one. That is exactly what happened; the resident proceeded to say that he and the other residents he knew were appalled that a baby they

viewed as having a dismal prognosis had been supported for so long. He resolved to speak with the attending that day. (ibid.:211).

The consequence was a rapid escalation of decision-making activity. Following conferences and consultations with specialists, a conference was held with the parents and it was unanimously decided to discontinue life support. While Anspach cannot be sure that this decision was the direct result of her intervention, she believes that, if she had remained silent, it would have been made much later.

Bosk (1992) describes a similar ethical dilemma, which arose in his observational study of genetic counseling but where he chose to remain silent, at the cost of some distress to himself. Either stance is potentially justifiable. What needs to be considered, though, is the quality of the reasoning that balances the moral responsibilities of citizenship and the integrity of science. Anspach leaned in one direction and Bosk in the other. Both provide their own justification on the facts of the case, which could not have been anticipated and determined by a prior scrutiny. To the extent that a judgment is made about their decisions, it is made by readers and reviewers after the event, rather than being open to an IRB in advance.

So far we have been concerned with the possibility that participants may be harmed, whether by a researcher's action or inaction, during the course of data collection. This corresponds with the period of maximum risk in biomedical experiments. In qualitative research, however, the period of risk can also extend beyond the completion of data collection. It is in the nature of both qualitative interviews and observational studies that researcher/participant relationships may go beyond the merely formal. The researcher's inevitable withdrawal at the end of the project can seem like loss or rejection (Patai 1991). Ironically, perhaps, the emphasis in feminist and similar standpoint research on trust, empathy, and nonhierarchical research relationships may actually increase this risk. Qualitative researchers need to give explicit attention to exit strategies that will minimize distress.

It is arguable that the most intractable problems arise when findings are published or delivered to commissioners (Cassell 1978; Wax & Cassell 1979). This is, of course, the very point at which researchers have least control. Once in the public domain, findings can be used for purposes that are at odds with the wishes of both researchers and research participants. It is here that the indeterminacy of the risks associated with qualitative research becomes most obvious (Patai 1991). Abrums (2000), for example, studied how the life experiences and belief systems of poor and working-class African-American women informed and influenced their opinions and interactions with the dominant white health care system. She recognized that, in spite of her commitment to feminist principles, there were limits to what she could do to control the uses to which the findings were put:

> I acknowledged that whatever I wrote could be used for political purposes to either hurt or to help black women and so I attempted to examine my writing carefully from every angle to see if it would contribute to the oppression of black women. (In the end I was not sure I could control how the reader would choose to use the information.) (ibid.:97)

Harm from the publication of qualitative research takes a number of different forms. First, there is the possibility that qualitative research may serve to expose practices and adaptive behaviors that research participants routinely use to resist institutional pressures of various kinds. Of course, this is very often exactly why a commissioner may want to contract for a qualitative study, taking advantage of its strengths in uncovering such information. However, commissioners need to think carefully about what they would do with the findings. The value of qualitative research to them may lie less in discovering that unauthorized behavior occurs—which is not exactly news—than in understanding why it happens and what it achieves for their institution. Simple attempts to neutralize or suppress unauthorized behavior risk being counterproductive if they actually subtract from the institution's efficiency or displace the behavior to somewhere more disruptive.

Some of these issues can be highlighted in McCorkel's (1998) study of a drug rehabilitation program for incarcerated female offenders, housed within a U.S. prison. This therapeutic community aimed to rehabilitate the women through a transformation of the self, achieved by a highly coercive control structure. Compared to the prison, the therapeutic community operated with "rules that are more restrictive, surveillance that is more pervasive, and punishments that are more severe" (ibid.:229). McCorkel described an intensive regime directed toward "breaking down" the addict through tight control of residents' actions and thoughts. It was explicitly structured to prevent residents forming alliances or supportive relationships with one another. Dress, demeanor, personal hygiene, movement within the facility, and facial expressions were all regulated. New residents were given a lengthy manual, which detailed permitted vocabulary and prohibited "street" language. This control was made possible through the elimination of private space. McCorkel describes the regime:

> In fact, there are no aspects of client's feelings, thoughts, or behaviors nor are there physical locations within the program facility that are not viewed as subject to surveillance and control. ... Staff not only control access to rooms, they also exert control over behavior within. ... Many incoming residents are

horrified when their roommates report to staff and other residents highly personal behaviors such as masturbation, poor hygiene, snoring, drooling, diarrhea, gas, vomiting, and crying. (ibid.:240)

McCorkel discovered that one small room, partly hidden in a corner of the building, was not subject to the same degree of surveillance:

> This room often serves as a forum for residents to critique the program and the counseling staff, and to express to other residents that they are not what the staff says they are. It is not a free place by Goffman's (1961) definition because counselors are thoroughly unaware of the subversive activities that are carried on in the room. (ibid.:242)

As long as staff remained unaware of how residents used this room, it represented a private space where residents could defend themselves against the regime. The secrecy of this activity was directly related to its usefulness to residents. By publishing details, McCorkel risked drawing staff attention to such "deviant" behavior and enabling them to prevent it. During her fieldwork McCorkel had deliberately distanced herself from the role of staff member in order to win residents' confidences. This had allowed her to gain insights into the residents' lives that would otherwise have been impossible:

> As my relationships with many of the PRW inmates grew increasingly friendly, they began to confide in me their doubts about the treatment program and, eventually, allowed me to be present when they evaded the surveillance of staff and discussed how best to survive the program. (ibid.:233)

McCorkel does not discuss the possible consequences, for the residents or their successors, of exposing their resistance strategies. By revealing the use to which residents put the "hidden room," McCorkel offered staff another mechanism by which to undermine the possibility of such resistance. Nor is it clear what this resistance achieves. Is it actually an important "safety valve" that makes the rest of the program possible by deflecting resident/staff confrontation? Are the discussions about survival between residents making a useful contribution to the therapeutic goals in unanticipated ways?

Second, the increasing pressure to disseminate research to "user audiences" means that findings often find their way into the mass media. The combination of human interest and health or disease is particularly attractive to journalists. However careful and respectful researchers are in their own writing, they can do little to prevent others presenting their findings in ways that cause offense or distress to study participants. This underlines researchers' obligations to protect participants' anonymity and to keep data confidential (Beauchamp 1993; Bulmer 1997). Such obligations are particularly difficult to observe in qualitative research because individual responses or behaviors cannot be lost within aggregated statistics. Much qualitative work is carried out in single settings or a small number of settings, making it more difficult to ensure that data are totally unattributable.

Qualitative researchers attempt to protect settings and participants by removing identifying information at the earliest possible opportunity, assigning pseudonyms, and altering nonrelevant details. However, none of these procedures can absolutely guarantee concealment. If fieldwork has been overt, many people will know that the research has been taking place and be able to identify the setting after publication. If the setting is relatively rare (such as, for example, a specialist tertiary care facility), the possibility of identification increases, particularly if the report contains reasonably detailed contextual information. Anspach (1993), for example, reports that she studied two intensive care nurseries in two different regions of the same state. She describes the first in considerable detail, using a pseudonym:

> Located in a demographically heterogeneous section of a large urban area, the Henry Maynard Randolph Hospital is part of a major medical school, is closely affiliated with a major university, and is commonly recognized as an elite institution. ... If neonatology may be characterized as medicine on the frontier, the Randolph Intensive-Care Nursery may be said to be on the frontier of that frontier. Several of its attending physicians are pioneers in the field, and discoveries made at the Randolph Nursery have become standard features in the armamentarium of contemporary neonatology. (ibid.:9)

Anspach goes on to describe the organizational hierarchy, staffing (including the educational qualifications of individual staff), and physical plant of the nursery in similar detail. She also gives information on the number of annual admissions, the sociodemographic profile of patients, and the financing of the facility. With this amount of information, a determined investigative journalist would find it relatively easy to identify the location. Certainly a number of cases have been reported where researchers' refusal to disclose their fieldwork site has not been sufficient to prevent journalists uncovering it (Morgan 1972; Lieblich 1996).

Where a research site is identified, participants face a range of risks. They may be publicly humiliated when aspects of their conduct and/or professional practices are exposed to public scrutiny. In some cases, they may even face investigation for possible professional or criminal offenses. As Anspach (1993) herself observed, the researcher may witness behaviors whose legal status is ambiguous, putting participants at risk of professional sanction, criminal prosecution, or civil suit if they are reported. Qualitative data have no legal immunity, although researchers may be able to derive some protection from the "shield laws" enacted in a few states, which allow journalists to refuse disclosure of confidential information during legal proceedings.

Third, even if researchers successfully protect the anonymity of research participants, studying particular places with particular groups of people who have ongoing lives and relationships inevitably makes it possible for participants to recognize themselves in publications (Richardson 1992). This is not always a comfortable experience. There is ample evidence that qualitative research reports can and do cause offense to those who are written about (Ellis 1995; Messenger 1989; Scheper-Hughes 1982; Vidich & Bensman 1958, 1964). Even when a research site remains anonymous to outsiders, participants are likely to be able to make educated guesses about the identities of others described in the research report. In his study of genetic counseling in a pediatric hospital, Bosk (1992) frequently reports the counselors' negative evaluations of the work of their neonatology colleagues. These reports usually refer to individual cases that are described in considerable detail. They are recorded *verbatim* and include allegations that the neonatologists were "shirking their responsibility," practicing "bad medicine," and "misallocating resources." These comments were invariably made after the doctor in question had left the room and it is doubtful whether the counselors intended that they should be fed back to the neonatologists in identifiable form. In his case, the situation was further complicated by the fact that he had been invited by the counseling team to study their work:

> To use a social analogy, I was often in the position of the guest invited to dinner where the experience of the meal itself is the entertainment—a feast. For this guest, nothing has been spared. The host has set the table with the best cutlery and china, given great attention to the menu, used the finest ingredients in preparing the dishes, and, nonetheless, produced an indifferent meal. ...
>
> On the one hand, I did not want to insult my hosts' hospitality. On the other, I did not want to respond enthusiastically to dismal fare, only to see it served up proudly on all occasions. What did I owe the genetic counselors as a result of the unique field opportunity that they afforded me? At one level, I felt that I owed it to them to present my criticisms at a very high level of generality, so that it was not individual counselors that I was criticizing, but the structural arrangements of care and the organization of social roles. (ibid.:11–12)

Bosk certainly does draw attention to structural arrangements and the organization of social roles in this book. However, in illustrating these points, he inevitably draws upon descriptions of the behaviors and interactions of individuals that are not always flattering or affirming.

Where researchers are attempting to do more than reproduce participant perspectives, it is likely that their analysis will disrupt some of the assumptions that participants make about their world and their actions within it (Borland 1991; Messenger 1989; Scheper-Hughes 1982). Encountering other versions of reality displayed in published texts may be a distressing experience. Lieblich described the most painful reaction to the publication of her work as

> that of family members who became aware, through the pages of the book, of memories, opinions and feelings that belonged to their family life and relationships that had never been discussed between them before. (1996:342)

Deciding what will or will not cause offense or distress is not always straightforward. Research participants may assume that research reports claim to represent some form of objective reality. They may be surprised if the research report does not affirm their own version of reality. Explaining that qualitative researchers treat any version of reality as just one of many possible versions may not reduce participants' sense of betrayal at the researcher's failure to accept and present their version as authoritative. The translation of individual experiences into examples of wider phenomena with the resulting loss of uniqueness may be disconcerting and people's views of themselves and their worlds may be deflated.

Respect for Persons

The second Belmont principle of "respect for persons" focuses on a rather different set of issues: the possibility that research subjects and participants may be wronged even when they are not harmed (MacIntyre 1982). Something that we take to be their right has been denied to them.

Traditionally, discussions about the rights of research participants have focused on autonomy and self-determination. This reflects the Nuremberg Code's insistence that the involvement of all human subjects in research must be voluntary and based upon adequate knowledge and understanding of the nature, duration, purpose, methods, and potential hazards of the study. It was the violation of this principle of "voluntary informed consent" that was at the heart of many of the criticisms of the Tuskegee (Jones 1981), Jewish Chronic Disease (Rothman 1993), and Willowbrook (Rothman 1993) studies introduced earlier in this chapter. The response to these abuses has been to place an obligation on biomedical researchers to obtain signed consent from research subjects who have been fully informed of the purpose, nature, methods, and potential risks of the study *in advance* of the their participation. Even in biomedical research, the use of signed consent forms is not unproblematic. In reality, they may offer more protection to the researcher than to the participants. Obtaining and retaining such forms may actually undermine participant anonymity by making the participants in a research study identifiable (Price 1996).

In spite of these difficulties, the practice of obtaining written consent from the subjects of biomedical experiments remains the lynchpin of codes of biomedical ethics. This emphasis is grounded in recognition of the power differential that exists between biomedical researchers and their subjects and well-founded outrage at its abuse in the notorious studies cited above. Written informed consent before any intervention remains the primary means of protecting the rights of research subjects. However, this is not always an appropriate, or indeed practical, safeguard in qualitative research.

First, there is a rather different power relationship between researchers and participants in qualitative and experimental research (Sheehan 1993). This applies particularly during data collection. Researcher power is intrinsic to experimental design (Cassell 1979). In giving consent, the research subject effectively surrenders the right to self-determination for the duration of the experiment. In qualitative research, participants have considerable capacity for exerting control over researchers (Hammersley 1992c; Wong 1998). Wong describes how he was rendered "helpless" during his study of how the New Jersey Welfare Reform Act (1991) impacted upon the domestic, sexual, productive, and reproductive lives of poor women enrolled in the Aid to Families with Dependent Children program:

> It is important to realize that the control often asserted by administrators and researchers is often illusionary. My respondents, in their desire to earn some extra cash to supplement their meager incomes, resisted and usurped the administrator's decisions on who should be chosen for the interviews. ... This created havoc and chaos in my scheduling and left me quite helpless. (1998:190)

Second, it is not always clear from whom one should seek written informed consent. Again this is generally straightforward in biomedical research, which typically involves the experimental treatment of individuals. Consent clearly has to be obtained from the individual subjects or their representatives. Qualitative interview studies can follow the same practice. Observational studies, however, may involve extended periods of work in semipublic settings such as hospital services or outpatient departments. Here the population is often highly transient and it is not always clear who should be classed as research participants. If the focus of observation is nurse behavior, should one seek consent not only from nurses but also from all the other people who are based on or even pass through the service? How far does this extend: to doctors? to cleaners? to patients? to visitors? to the catering assistants who bring the food trolleys round? Even if one does negotiate the consent of all these different individuals at the outset of a study, is one then obliged formally to renegotiate each time there is a change of personnel or patients?

Bosk's (1992) study of genetic counseling illustrates some of these complexities. As we have noted, Bosk was invited to carry out the research by the counselors who were its focus. Their participation can clearly be defined as voluntary and consensual. However, they were not the only people to come within Bosk's sphere of observation. Indeed, much of his analysis deals with the interactions between counselors, pediatricians, and parents. Bosk describes his own initial lack of awareness of the ethical issues that this raised:

> I also never stopped to worry that some of the data might have been gathered unethically. After all, I sometimes lacked fully informed, voluntary consent. While genetic counselors volunteered for study, other pediatricians were observed without their knowledge, as were patients; when consulting, there sometimes was not ample opportunity to introduce the ethnographer. If opportunity existed, it was hard to imagine at the time how the introduction would help a troubled situation. (ibid.:161–62)

In some cases, researchers appear to treat consent as a practical rather than an ethical issue. Typically they only seek consent from those who have the power to control their access. Fujimoto (2001) describes how she negotiated access to a therapeutic community for teen mothers with the project director but made no attempt to seek permission from the women taking part in the program. Indeed, at the director's suggestion, she did not disclose her identity as a researcher for the first month of the study. Although she later did tell the women of her purpose, she does not appear to have felt that it was appropriate to seek their permission. She herself comments on the way in which this failure to seek consent from the participants reflected "the power dynamics of the setting" in which "the group had no say in who would witness their therapy" (ibid.:4). Strangely, Fujimoto appears to treat this as a criticism of the program but does not reflect upon her own responsibility.

Third, there is the problem of the *adequacy* of participants' knowledge of the nature, duration, methods, and potential hazards of the research, as envisaged by the Nuremberg Code. The definition of "adequate" is not straightforward. Much research, whether biomedical or social scientific, is embedded in highly technical theoretical constructs. It can be difficult to provide an accessible explanation without distorting the research's true nature. The versions that we offer to research participants are necessarily designed for the audiences to which they are directed. If that were not so they might well be true but they would be incomprehensible.

This difficulty is shared by both conventional biomedical and qualitative research. In experimental research, though, the nature of the study is normally determined in advance, so that participants can be fully briefed. The design and focus of qualitative studies are more likely to evolve in the course of the research so that the risks are less determinate and easily characterized in advance. It is often impossible to give informants a complete account of the nature of a study from the beginning simply because the investigator may not be entirely certain where it is going.

For example, in the research referred to earlier, Voysey (1975) initially intended that the outcome would be a description of the problems facing families with a disabled child, which would lead to improvements in health and social care services. She negotiated access to her informants on this basis. However, in the course of the study, the focus of her research was transformed. She began to realize that her interview data were best understood as a set of accounts where parents felt constrained to present themselves as "good parents." In her book, Voysey presents a compelling and sensitive analysis of the moral worlds in which such families function. However, it bears little resemblance to the study outcomes that formed the basis of her initial negotiations with parents. In that sense, one could not claim that she had fully informed consent for the study that she actually carried out.

Even where the researcher is clear about the likely nature and outcomes of a piece of research from the outset, this does not mean that he or she is able to communicate these to the participants. This may be because the participants have preconceptions about the research that influence their interpretation of whatever information the researcher offers. Such notions may be unexpressed and therefore not open to challenge or refutation by the researcher. Once again, this is well illustrated by Bosk's study of genetic counseling. Bosk describes how he came to realize that the access he was granted by genetic counselors in a pediatric clinic was based upon an assumption that he would act as a "committed moral entrepreneur, [who would provide] society at large with data that would confirm the need to commit an even greater supply of resources to genetic counseling" (1992:6).

This assumption was not based upon any statement of intention from Bosk. Rather, he suggests,

> The genetic counselors believed that such a commitment was necessary and that, if I came to know their world as they did, I too would find such a need inescapable. This expectation—that our sentiments and analyses of societal interest would prove to be congruent—was, of course, unstated at the outset. It came with the invitation, but I did not realize it at the time. (ibid.:6–7)

Clearly the consent of these genetic counselors was not fully informed but, given the impenetrability of the counselors' preconceptions, it is difficult to see how it could have been otherwise.

For all these reasons, the insistence upon signed consent forms for all qualitative research appears to be an inadequate and inappropriate means of ensuring the autonomy of participants in qualitative research studies. This is not to suggest that the principle of informed consent is irrelevant. It is, rather, to argue that the ritual of obtaining a signature on a consent form is an inadequate guarantee that the rights of research participants are properly protected. Genuine protection comes from the researcher's ongoing commitment throughout the research process and willingness to withdraw, amend, or constrain the emergent research design whenever there is irresolvable conflict with the wishes of the research participants. The rights of participants in qualitative research are protected more by the moral sense of the researcher than by the prescriptive rules or rituals of regulatory codes.

Most qualitative researchers interpret respect for persons as requiring observational work to be carried out as overtly as possible without causing disruption or distress in the setting. A minority, however, reject the principle of informed consent entirely, justifying the use of covert observational methods. In such studies, the researcher may even deliberately mislead participants about his or her true reason for participating in a setting. Covert observation often seems superficially attractive in enhancing the validity of qualitative work by reducing its impact on a setting to the absolute minimum (Homan 1980). The ends that it achieves are held to justify the means, particularly where access might otherwise be difficult or denied, and the potential for harm is considered insignificant.

There are a number of well-known examples, of which the most famous, or possibly infamous, is Laud Humphreys's (1970) study of sexual encounters between homosexual men in public lavatories. This study, published under the title *Tearoom Trade*, involved periods of observation where Humphreys played the role of "watch-queen" or lookout for men engaged in homosexual acts that were, at that time, illegal. He then traced the men, using their car registration numbers, and carried out research interviews with them, in their own homes, posing as an interviewer in an anonymous health survey. Humphreys's work provoked considerable controversy, particularly over his tracing of the men, which created risks for them, in a more conservative era, of criminal prosecution, family breakdown, and social stigmatization.

In spite of this barrage of criticism, some qualitative researchers have continued to defend the use of covert methods. Timothy Diamond's (1992) observational study of nursing homes in Chicago involved a significant amount of covert research. Diamond underwent a six-month training as a nursing assistant and then worked in three different nursing homes for periods of three to four months. Initially, he had intended to disclose his research purposes at every phase of the study. In fact, in the early stages, he did reveal his role to some of his fellow nursing staff and to some residents. However, Diamond reports that, "as the study proceeded it was forced increasingly to become a piece of undercover research" (ibid.:8). Diamond feared that if his employers came to know about the research he would be sacked. He would not have lied if he had been asked a direct question about his researcher role. However, this situation did not arise and his identity was kept secret from the managers and administrators of the homes he worked in. He justifies this by claiming that he would have been unable to complete the study if he had disclosed his true purposes:

> Though I had not intended to be secretive, the situations left me no choice. When I said I wanted to do research no one hired me. (ibid.:247)

Diamond's position appears to be that the value of his research in exposing the exploitation of nursing assistants and the erosion of patient autonomy, privacy, and dignity outweighs any wrong done. The outcome justifies the means used. This is always a risky argument because it leaves the researcher as the final arbiter of who has or has not the right to autonomy and self-determination. If the Belmont principles have any meaning, then respect for persons is indivisible: managers have rights too.

Even if we accept Diamond's argument in relation to the powerful within the settings he studied, we are still left with the problem of the less powerful. Many of the nursing assistants and residents were also deceived by Diamond. Although he does not say so, this was presumably because requesting their permission to record and write about their daily lives would have increased the risk of his identity being exposed to home managements. It is somewhat ironic that, as a consequence, Diamond himself reproduces many of the wrongs he claims are done to the residents and nursing staff by the management. He has penetrated their privacy, in the role of nursing assistant, and publicizes their humiliation and loss of dignity without having secured their consent. His motivation for doing so is entirely honorable. He is obviously committed to righting the wrongs he observed. However, in doing so he has compromised both their autonomy and their dignity.

The mainstream view in qualitative research, however, is cool or hostile to the use of covert methods. The outcomes of covert research are not the only criterion by which it should be judged (Dingwall 1980; Beauchamp, Faden, & Wallace 1982). The difficulties of obtaining valid data using overt methods can be exaggerated (Dingwall 1980). Researchers have been granted open access to highly sensitive settings and groups including the British Civil Service (Heclo & Wildavsky 1974), the Mafia (Ianni & Ianni 1972), professional "fences" (Klockars 1979), professional criminals (Polsky 1971), and drug barons (Adler 1985). Covert researchers may well underestimate the harm that their studies may cause. As we saw in the last section, people do read what we write and, in the case of covert research, a sense of betrayal may be intensified where the people we study discover that we have misled them about the true nature of our interest in them (Bulmer 1980). Above all, covert research involves invading the privacy of those we study and denying their right to autonomy and self-determination.

However open the research agenda, though, the prolonged contact characteristic of qualitative research may mean that, in time, participants overlook the reason for the researcher's presence. This can happen to a limited extent in qualitative interviews if the informant begins to treat the interviewer as a friend or confidant. It is even more likely in a participant observation study where the researcher becomes fully integrated into the research setting. Such integration is often seen as the mark of a skilled researcher, minimizing reactivity and increasing confidence that the data collected are not distorted by his or her presence. However, it also poses problems. Murray (2000) describes some of the complexities that arose in the course of four and a half years' fieldwork in two child-care centers. She was appointed as an administrator to the two centers. Both the teachers and the directors knew, before hiring her, that she was doing research on child-care workers. She explained that the research would involve interviews and observation and that she would be taking fieldnotes during the course of her work. To that extent, one could claim that Murray had negotiated "informed consent." However, as she herself remarks, the center staff did not always appear to be conscious of her research role as she interacted with them. Murray became privy to a great deal of confidential "insider information" in the course of her work. She describes the dilemma she faced: "How much should I tell workers about my observations and how often should I tell them?" (ibid.:140).

She chose not to remind the workers that she was doing research each time they entered her office and avoided taking notes in front of them. It is clear that Murray was not entirely comfortable with this decision. In particular, she felt compromised when she crossed what she describes as "the indefinable line into friendship" with some of the workers and, at that point, chose to stop taking notes.

Safeguarding the rights of participants in qualitative research is far from straightforward. It is complicated by a number of issues, including the emergent nature of the research design, the complex nature of research settings, and the prolonged periods of time that researchers often spend collecting data. These factors mean that reliance upon obtaining signed consent at the outset of the study is usually misplaced. To be meaningful, the negotiation of informed consent for qualitative research needs to continue throughout the study. It depends on the researcher's commitment to protecting the rights of research participants even where this may mean compromises in relation to research design.

Justice

In research on health care, there is always a danger that the perspective of professionals will dominate. Patient understandings, perspectives, and preferences are often treated as defective versions of those held by professionals. The implicit or explicit agenda of the research becomes that of identifying patients' shortcomings and ways in which these can be "corrected." Researchers are frequently warned against adopting this kind of deferential posture and encouraged to ensure that they do justice to the perspectives of the less powerful members of the settings they study (Guba & Lincoln 1989; Marshall 1985; Sandelowski 1986).

Much qualitative research is now explicitly committed to adopting the so-called underdog perspective, a commitment to speak for the oppressed and exploited (see Chapter 1). This appears to be the position adopted by Diamond (1992). He is committed to describing the everyday life of residents in nursing homes, and of the frontline staff who care for them, from their own perspective. In doing so, he paints a disturbing picture of the officiousness, inflexibility, and inhumanity of the home administrators. His exposure of the indignities and abuses that make up the daily lives of residents and frontline staff is not balanced with any attempt to understand the world in which the administrators operate or the conditions that hold their behaviors in place. The methodological implications of this "underdog perspective" are taken up in the next chapter. However, this approach does also raise questions of justice.

Diamond's treatment of the nursing home administrators echoes Bosk's description of the approach most sociologists take to the medical profession (Bosk 1992). Bosk suggests that sociologists tend to see the medical profession as

> a living breathing exemplar of G. B. Shaw's "conspiracy against the laity." The sociologist's task is to expose this conspiracy for what it is—the exploitation of pain and vulnerability for profit. (ibid.:5)

Bosk, by contrast, saw his goal as one of describing the practice of genetic counseling, identifying "the embedded tensions that lie beneath the surface of a rapidly advancing and dazzling medical technology" (ibid.:18). As such he was committed to understanding the ways in which the counselors' practices were held in place. While sympathetic to the difficulties and constraints under which genetic counselors operate, Bosk's account of their practice is far from uncritical. He is careful to examine "the shadow that falls between the image and reality" (ibid.) of genetic counseling practice. As such his account preserves a critical distance from the practices of those he studies without reducing their behavior to the impenetrable machinations of Machiavellian villains.

The principle of justice requires qualitative researchers to treat all those they study evenhandedly. This does not, of course, mean that researchers are obliged to suspend all personal moral judgment. Rather it requires them to pursue a systematically disinterested approach (Oakley 1998) to the phenomena under investigation. It demands that they commit themselves to developing an equally sophisticated understanding of the behavior of all members of the settings they study and the perspectives of all those whom they interview (Dingwall 1992).

CONCLUSION

In this chapter, we have explored some of the complex ethical issues that arise in the conduct of qualitative research and that should be of concern to commissioners, practitioners, and consumers of research. We have suggested that the same ethical principles apply to qualitative and biomedical research. However, the differences between research practices of the two traditions are such that the application of these principles to the design and conduct of research is somewhat different in each case. The implementation of risk-benefit analysis and the practice of obtaining written informed consent are inadequate and, in some cases, inappropriate responses to the ethical dilemmas thrown up in qualitative research studies. Ethical qualitative research practice will not be guaranteed through the imposition of a prescriptive list of requirements or the ritualized administration of consent forms. Rather it depends upon the conscientious and reflective commitment of individual researchers and research teams to identifying and minimizing any potential harm to participants, to negotiating fully informed consent not only at the outset but also throughout the research process, and to treating all those under study with disinterested even-handedness. There is clearly a major challenge in ensuring both that IRBs are aware of the extent of their discretion, and have the confidence to use it, and that qualitative researchers are adequately trained in order to sustain IRB confidence.

NOTES

1. As Hazelgrove (2002) notes, recent studies have also questioned some of the research done by the Allies on their own soldiers and civilians during World War

II. The Allies were quick to set up a commission to consider what scientific lessons could be learned from the concentration camp work and to reemploy those doctors who were not included in the trial but had relevant knowledge.

2. This account is based on the Introduction to Penslar and Porter (1993). See http://ohrp.osophs.dhhs.gov/irb/irdb_introduction.htm.

3. See, for example, the hearing of the National Human Research Protection Advisory Committee (NHRPAC) on January 29, 2002 (Church 2002).

4. Qualitative researchers normally use pseudonyms for participants in their research. Timmermans had neglected to include the conventional footnote about this and IRB members had thought they were seeing real names.

5. These principles reflect the assumptions of postwar U.S. liberalism about the rights of the individual, the virtues of self-determination, and the nature of justice (Benatar 1997). They are not universals (Christians 2000). They tend to give primacy to individual rights over collective interests to a degree that other societies find questionable (Wolpe 1998). Although U.S. bioethics has been a major customer for qualitative research, as a contribution to its debates over clinical practice, we shall not specifically discuss that body of work here (see Bosk 2000). The methodological issues that arise in that context are generic ones and merely require the application of the arguments that we set out in reviewing the full range of applications of qualitative research. It should also be noted that bioethicists involved in debates over clinical practice have become increasingly critical of the principlist approach, although it remains more central to debates over research ethics.

6. The complex relationship between interview accounts and informants' experiences is discussed in Chapter 5.

III

Evaluating
Qualitative Research

9

Judging the Quality of Qualitative Research

In this chapter we consider how the quality of qualitative research can and should be judged. This issue is of prime significance to both commissioners and consumers of qualitative health-related research, whether they are policymakers, practitioners, or academics. It takes us back to the substance of Chapter 1, where we discussed the heterogeneity of the qualitative research tradition. We saw there that the field of qualitative research is characterized by radical disagreements about the purpose, assumptions, and practice of qualitative research. Not surprisingly, these disagreements are reflected in claims and counterclaims about how the products of such research activity should be assessed. The question of appropriate criteria for assessing qualitative research is closely related to the question of the appropriate and legitimate goals of such research, and it is to this issue that we first turn our attention.

BY WHAT CRITERIA SHOULD WE JUDGE QUALITATIVE RESEARCH?

In Chapter 1, we noted that some qualitative researchers actively reject science, with its commitment to the search for authoritative knowledge, as an appropriate model for their research. This immediately calls into question the appropriateness of conventional scientific criteria such as validity and reliability for judging research outputs. In turn, this has given rise to discussion about what alternative criteria might fit better with the antirealist and relativist assumptions that some argue are central to qualitative research practice.

In fact, some writers, such as John Smith (1984), argue against the whole notion of criteria for assessing qualitative research. Smith contends that since people "may construct their realities in their own different ways at different times and places" (ibid.:382) it is nonsense to identify some versions of reality as trustworthy and others not. He argues that relativists who seek to develop criteria for judging qualitative research are attempting the impossible:

> The assumptions of multiple realities and reality as mind-involved seriously undermine the notion of applying foundational criteria to distinguish trustworthy results from untrustworthy ones. The assumptions and foundational criteria are, in a word, incompatible. ... Different claims about reality result not from incorrect procedures but may simply be a case of one investigator's reality versus another's. (ibid.:383)

Smith's argument is logically unassailable. If we accept his premise (that there are potentially as many realities as there are persons) then his conclusion (that there are no grounds on which we might judge the relative trustworthiness of research outputs) follows inexorably. However, such a conclusion will be unacceptable to most research commissioners and research consumers. It undermines the potential usefulness of research for informing the organization and delivery of health care. Smith's position is also profoundly uncomfortable for researchers who seek relevance to policy and practice. If no standards can legitimately be applied to qualitative research, or to its products, why would we expect policymakers and practitioners to attend to them, far less act upon them? As Altheide and Johnson have argued,

> As long as we strive to base our claims and interpretations of social life on data of any kind, we must have a logic for assessing and communicating the interactive processes through which the investigator acquired the research experience and information. (1994:485)

Not all researchers who share Smith's antirealist assumptions abandon the possibility of establishing criteria for judging qualitative research. More often they argue that, since qualitative research is a distinctive paradigm, criteria such as validity and reliability, imported from the "dominant" quantitative or positivist paradigm, are inappropriate. They offer instead a range of alternative criteria, which are seen as more relevant to the qualitative "paradigm." The result has been an explosion of novel concepts and criteria for judging qualitative research. Some of these seek to qualify the conventional notion of validity in some way. Altheide and Johnson report finding all the following variations on this term: "successor validity, catalytic validity, interrogated validity, transgressive validity, imperial validity, simulcra/ironic validity, situated validity and voluptuous validity"

(Altheide & Johnson 1994: 488). Others introduce new criteria such as "credibility," "transferability," "dependability," and "confirmability" (Lincoln & Guba 1985: 488), or "structural corroboration," "referential adequacy," and "multiplicative replication" (Eisner 1983:13-14). To the extent that such attempts to formulate alternatives to conventional criteria are antirealist they are inherently contradictory. On the one hand, they seek to establish some basis for judging the trustworthiness of research findings. On the other, they embrace a version of relativism in which the world is characterized by "multiple constructed realities." As Seale has commented, "Relativism does not sit well with attempts to establish truth, even if the term is placed in inverted commas" (1999:46).

In Chapter 1 we also discussed versions of qualitative research that erode the boundaries between research and politics, embracing emancipation from sources of domination and oppression as their primary goal. This is reflected in the criteria proposed for judging such work. Conventional criteria are criticized for obscuring the political function of research reports by presenting findings as neutral and authoritative. These writers seek to establish overtly political criteria for research. Validity is once again either redefined or abandoned as an appropriate criterion. For example, Roman and Apple (1990) argue that validity should be defined in terms of the extent to which studies are democratically designed and the results democratically produced. The extent of democratization can, they argue, be established using four measures:

1. The extent to which the study resonates with the "lived experience" of those being researched.
2. The extent to which the study enables members of the group being studied to comprehend and transform their experiences of subordination.
3. The extent to which the study reduces the divide between the researcher's intellectual work and the group members' ordinary ways of describing and understanding their experiences.
4. The extent to which the research allows the researcher's prior and political commitments to be informed and transformed by understandings derived from the group's experiences. (ibid.:63–64)

Similarly Mies (1983) redefines validity in terms of the research's contribution to emancipation. She argues that "the 'truth' of a theory is not dependent on the application of certain methodological principles and rules, but on its potential to orient the processes of praxis towards progressive emancipation and humanization" (ibid.:124).

As we showed in Chapter 1, not all qualitative researchers embrace relativism. Nor do they necessarily treat research as a form of political action. Indeed there are both principled and pragmatic reasons for refusing to do either. The subtle realist position we outlined marries a recognition that both empirical observations and theoretical inferences are always and irreducibly influenced by the frame of references and assumptions we bring to the study, in this case the recognition that the phenomena we are studying have a reality that is independent of our observations. While it is perfectly possible to have multiple different representations of the same phenomena, not all representations are equally likely to be true. This opens up the possibility of judging the likely truth or otherwise of research findings. Of course, such judgments are always provisional and we cannot ever reach a position of absolute certainty about truth claims. Further evidence may cast doubt upon findings we once judged to be secure. All knowledge claims depend upon assumptions, the validity of which we take as given, at least for the present (Hammersley 1990).

Judgments about the quality of research findings relate to the extent to which claims are supported by convincing evidence. In particular, we are concerned with how far error has been limited in the design, analysis, and reporting of research. As Hammersley observes, this relatively modest notion of truth as "beliefs about whose validity we are reasonably confident" (1992a:50) is not confined to qualitative research:

> I believe that we can *never* be certain about the truth of anything, not even in the natural sciences or in our personal lives. On the other hand, there are many things about whose truth we are very confident and about which we have every right to be confident. (1990:59, emphasis in original)

HOW CAN WE ASSESS THE TRUTH CLAIMS OF QUALITATIVE RESEARCH?

There are no simple algorithmic criteria by which the truth claims of qualitative research can be assessed. Such assessments always involve judgments grounded in evidence. Both researchers and consumers of research findings have responsibilities for making such judgments. Researchers have a double responsibility here. First, they have a responsibility for rigorous and self-critical conduct, analysis, and interpretation of the research. It is by the systematic and relentless search for contradictory evidence that error is limited and the claim to authoritative knowledge is strengthened. Second, they have a responsibility to present the readers of research with sufficient information to allow the latter to decide whether their proposed findings are adequately supported. This leads on to the responsibilities of research consumers. It is for them to make an evidence-based judgment about the likely truth of research findings, taking into account the efforts the researchers have made to limit error during the research process. This involves a judgment about the soundness of the evidence base on which those claims are made and a consideration of possible alternative interpretations of the data obtained.

Research reports can be treated as authoritative when we are convinced that the possibility of error has been limited to the greatest extent possible. A search for disconfirming evidence is central to claims that error has been limited. We will be more convinced of the truth of a claim when there is evidence that the researchers have exposed their ideas and analyses to rigorous attempts at refutation before they are presented to the research audience.

A number of procedures for hunting down contradictory evidence have been proposed and these are discussed below. However, it is important to recognize that generating confidence in the truth of one's research findings is not "simply a matter of finding and following certain analytic procedures" (Phillips 1987:21). There is a risk that such procedures turn into rigid constraints that become ends in themselves rather than enhancing the validity of the research. Moreover, since most research is resource-limited, it typically involves trade-offs between various approaches to enhancing the validity of the study and budgetary and other practical constraints.

SEARCHING FOR CONTRADICTORY EVIDENCE

It is both impossible and, indeed, largely undesirable for qualitative researchers to approach their empirical work *tabula rasa*. As we have argued throughout this book, observations are necessarily impregnated with prior assumptions and references, whether or not researchers are able or willing to articulate these. Increasingly, also, qualitative research is informed by previous empirical studies carried out in similar settings. All of this means that researchers approach their task with resources drawn from their own personal and academic autobiographies and from their reading of the relevant literature. Moreover, as researchers begin to collect data, whether through observations, documents, or interviews, they will begin to notice patterns and to draw conclusions about "what is going on here." This can be a particularly fruitful period since their novice status often means that researchers notice things which, with greater familiarity, they would simply take for granted as natural or inevitable.

Both sets of ideas—the initial ones researchers bring to their empirical work and those generated in early fieldwork—can be very valuable. However, they also carry dangers. As Sandelowski (1986) argues, "holistic bias" is a major threat to the validity of qualitative research. By this she is referring to the tendency of some qualitative researchers to make their data look more patterned than they really are. Preliminary ideas can act as a filter through which researchers see the phenomena under study and the data they collect. As a result, they are alert to evidence that confirms their prior assumptions and fail to notice data that contradicts or modifies these preliminary ideas. This can lead to research reports that do not go beyond the presentation of interesting ideas, supported by illustrative quotes from the data.

Bosk reflects upon the risk of overgeneralizing from individual events and the means by which he sought to overcome this temptation in his study of surgical mistakes:

> There is the danger that one particular event will become etched in the field-worker's memory as emblematic of the way action is organized in an environment. That is to say that field-workers may overgeneralize incidents and see them as representative of categories of action. ... I avoided overgeneralization by making sure I had at least two independently generated examples of the same phenomenon before I began to make inferences. My operating rule here was, as far as I can see, not fundamentally different than those that survey researchers use to ensure reliability in their studies. Also, I was very careful to follow particular incidents through many levels of social organization. For example, I was able to test my inferences about normative error in the promotion meeting, where I observed the criteria attending surgeons use to judge the fitness of housestaff for surgical careers. Throughout my fieldwork, I was very careful to test observations in one context against those of another. (1979:207)

One of the defining characteristics of high-quality qualitative research is a rigorous and systematic search for evidence that contradicts or modifies the emerging analysis. This can take many forms at different stages of the research project. First, the search for negative evidence can be the underlying rationale for an entire study. This is an important way in which qualitative research contributes to the accumulation of knowledge in a particular field. For example, Markens and colleagues (Markens, Browner, & Press 1999) interviewed Californian women who refused prenatal screening for alpha-fetoprotein (AFP). Previous research focused upon women who participate in the screening program and had concluded that the program was yet another example of the "infiltration of physicians and medical technologies into the reproductive process" (ibid.:360). Little research had been conducted upon women who refused AFP: this study was designed to fill that gap.

The researchers approached this study with the expectation that women who refused AFP were either opposed to abortion (the only medical intervention available after a positive test) or were actively resisting both medicalization and the definition of their pregnancies in biomedical terms. In fact, the data collected challenged these assumptions. AFP refusal did not reflect rejection of or resistance to biomedicine and technology. Indeed many of the women actively drew upon the logic of biomedicine to defend their refusal of AFP. They formulated this refusal in terms of the potential risks of the test—all risks that were framed in biomedical terms. Indeed they found more similarities than differences between those who accepted and those who refused the test when their views toward abortion and biomedicine were compared.

A second example of openness to revision of prior assumptions is found in Steven Taylor's (2000) study of a family (the Dukes) all of whose members have been officially defined as handicapped, disabled, or "retarded." Taylor approached this study informed by both his reading of the sociological and anthropological literature on disability and stigma and his own previous ethnographic study of a ward at Empire State School, an "institution for the mentally retarded." Previous research suggested that people who were classified as retarded would experience this label as profoundly humiliating and stigmatizing and would actively resist and reject the associated moral identity. The life histories he carried out with former residents of Empire State School again suggested that people would avoid volunteering that they had lived in such an institution. It was, therefore, something of a surprise to Taylor when Bill, the father of the Dukes family, introduced himself as a "graduate of Empire State School." This alerted Taylor to the possibility that his own assumptions, and those in the literature, that those labeled as "retarded" could not maintain a positive identity, were mistaken. Through a detailed analysis of the Dukes' interactions within their family and friendship networks and with formal organizations, Taylor identified some of the factors that accounted for the Dukes' ability to avoid the stigma and spoiled identities generally associated with disability. He uses this family as a critical case to suggest ways in which the claims derived from previous studies of disability and stigma might usefully be modified.

In both these cases, confidence in the trustworthiness of the analyses is enhanced by evidence that assumptions drawn from previous studies have been subjected to empirical test and modified in the light of subsequent findings. The same commitment to hunting down contradictory evidence can be found within individual studies. For example, another study of people with a diagnosis of mental retardation (Edgerton 1967), which was introduced in Chapter 6, is notable for its attention to including in the analysis all the cases studied. Edgerton interviewed and carried out participant observation among forty-eight ex-patients of a large state institution for the mentally retarded. All were now living in the community and Edgerton explored how they managed their lives and perceived themselves. Edgerton is careful to make it clear when a claim he makes on the basis of his data applies to the whole sample. For example, he reports that one of the first challenges the ex-patients faced was concealing that they had been in an institution for the mentally retarded. In practice, they dealt with this challenge by developing a stereotyped story that revealed the "real" reason they were there. Edgerton confirms that "such excuses were collected from all of the forty-eight ex-patients" (ibid.:148). He then goes on to present examples of the different kinds of excuses found within his data. The authority of Edgerton's claim is strengthened by his systematic search of his whole dataset for cases that might contradict his claim, rather than relying upon a few readily available data extracts for support. That he found no contradictory cases increases our confidence in his findings. However, this is also an example of the provisional nature of even the most rigorously developed claims. Taylor's subsequent study of the Dukes family, which was introduced above, identified at least one case in which a person with a history of attending a state institution for the mentally retarded did not make recourse to excuses in the way in which Edgerton reported (Taylor 2000). This underlines the observation we made earlier that all claims to knowledge, however well supported by data, are subject to reappraisal in the light of further evidence.

The conscientious search for negative evidence does sometimes turn up cases that challenge the emerging analysis. When this happens, the researcher has the opportunity to modify the analysis to take account of the negative cases. This is an important means by which the analysis of qualitative findings can be refined so that it becomes more sensitive to the full range of data. An example of such modification in the light of negative evidence is found in Gubrium and Buckholdt's (1982) analysis of the social organization of care in a rehabilitation hospital, which was discussed in Chapter 6.

Within this hospital, support groups were organized by staff for the families of patients. There were separate support groups for the families of stroke patients and for those of patients with spinal cord injuries. Gubrium and Buckholdt observed that the emphasis in the two groups was very different. In the spinal injury group, staff stressed the importance of full independence and, in particular, being able to live separately from their families. The families were encouraged to embrace this goal as being in the best interests of the patient, even where the patients themselves did not aspire to live independently. By contrast, the ideal future promoted for stroke patients was much more closely tied to the family. Independent living was interpreted very differently for this group and was seen as being critically dependent upon family support.

The researchers found that this difference in the way in which the "ideal future" was conceptualized in the two groups held irrespective of actual physical condition. However, they identified a small number of cases in which this generalization did not apply. In these cases, either independent living was stressed for stroke patients or those with spinal cord injuries were presented as needing intensive support from their families. Detailed examination of these cases showed that they differed from others within their particular support group in terms of the patient's age. In cases where independence was presented as important for stroke victims, the patients were found to be considerably younger than most patients in that group. Similarly, in cases where the need for family support was stressed for spinal cord injury patients, the patients were found to be elderly. In the light of this superficially contradictory evidence, Gubrium and Buckholdt concluded that the critical factor in determining whether independence or dependence was promoted was not the patient's particular diagnosis but their age. It was simply the case that most stroke patients were elderly and most spinal cord patients were young. The authors sum up their conclusions:

> These exceptions support the age rule: "When a stroke patient is unusually young, the view of limited hope for strokes is not considered applicable; it still applies however to 'common' strokes. When a cord-injured person is old, the view of limitless hope again does not apply, for the same reason." (ibid.:115)

Seale's (1995) study of the accounts given by the relatives of people who died alone, which was discussed in detail in Chapter 5, again shows how the incorporation of negative data can strengthen the analysis. From his analysis of the accounts given by 149 relatives and friends of people who had died alone, Seale concluded that these accounts were all concerned to repair the informants' identity as members of a caring community in the face of the challenge posed by such unaccompanied death. As already discussed, the majority stressed that they had been eager to accompany the person who died and that their failure to do so was the result of some mishap. However, Seale did find five accounts where informants denied that they had wanted to be present when their relative/friend died. Rather than simply dismissing these as insignificant outliers, Seale subjected these five cases to detailed analysis. In all five cases, he was able to show how their failure to be present when their friend/relative died was nevertheless presented as compatible with their membership of a caring moral community.

In the examples we have just described, the identification and analysis of negative cases is, to some extent, incidental or serendipitous. The researchers have identified a general pattern in their data and then have subjected the entire dataset to systematic analysis to confirm or deny the universality of that pattern. In doing so, they uncovered some "negative cases" that appeared to challenge their emergent analysis, leading to its modification. However, as we saw in Chapter 6, it is also possible to build the search for contradictory evidence into the research design itself.

The analysis of qualitative data typically takes place alongside the data collection. This opens up further possibilities for the search for negative evidence. In the course of preliminary data analysis, the researcher produces some tentative generalizations. The interplay between data collection and analysis creates the conditions under which those tentative generalizations can be subjected to empirical testing. To do so, the researcher systematically looks for situations under which those generalizations are least likely to hold. For example, if researchers have observed certain patterns of interaction between doctors and nurses during daytime shifts on a surgical ward, they might choose to carry out further observations to discover whether those same patterns occur during nighttime shifts. Similarly, they could decide to observe nonsurgical wards to discover whether the tentative generalizations hold in other specialties. The ways in which these kinds of sampling strategies were adopted by both Glaser and Strauss (1965b, 1967) and Bosk (1979) were examined in Chapter 6. As we also saw in Chapter 6, through the example of Guillemin and Holmstrom's (1986) study of pediatric intensive care, the search for negative evidence can take the researchers far beyond the original research site.

In this section, we have examined some of the many ways in which qualitative researchers can demonstrate their commitment to limiting error in the claims they make on the basis of their data through systematic and conscientious searching for contradictory data. We do not suggest that all of these methods should be applied within every single study. This is not a checklist of dos and don'ts. Rather, we have illustrated a range of ways in which a commitment to searching for contradictory evidence can be operationalized. In the next two sections, we expand on this theme in relation to, first, the use of a variety of methods within research studies and, second, the exposure of one's analysis to feedback from research participants.

COMBINING DIFFERENT METHODS

As we have seen in previous chapters, qualitative data can be obtained using a variety of methods, including observation, interviews, interaction analysis, and documentary analysis. Qualitative methods can be combined with quantitative data collection, either within a single study or in a linked series of studies. There is no such thing as a perfect research method. All methods involve trade-offs and some methods are better for some purposes than for others. Decisions about which methods to use in particular circumstances to address particular research goals are essentially pragmatic. A key concern in judging the quality of the research is the appropriateness of the methods selected to answer the question at hand. In other words, "Are the methods used in this study fit for the purpose to which they have been put?"

Some research questions can be answered adequately using a single method. For example, if we are concerned with the nature of doctor-patient interactions in a specific setting, some form of interaction analysis may be perfectly adequate. However, if we wish to understand how contextual factors impact upon such interactions, we may wish to combine interaction analysis with observational data. Similarly, if we wish to discover how patients talk about their consultations with doctors, interview data will be adequate for our purposes. On the other hand, if our aim is to relate such descriptions to what actually happens within doctor-patient consultations, some combination of interviews and observation or interaction analysis will be required. The combination of several methods within a single study can be an important means of limiting error. It can do this in a number of ways.

First, using a variety of methods can limit error by increasing the comprehensiveness of a study and thus the likelihood that negative evidence will be uncovered. Renee Anspach's (1993) study of life-and-death decisions in two intensive care nurseries demonstrates this. Her primary method was observational. She spent a total of sixteen months observing in two intensive care nurseries. Her focus upon just one relatively rare feature of such nurseries (life-and-death decisions) created some difficulties insofar as many such decisions are made at impromptu conferences. Since Anspach could not be present in the nursery all of the time, it was inevitable that some of the decisions she was interested in were made in her absence. Over time, as she became familiar with the culture of the nursery, Anspach became skilled in anticipating when such a decision was looming and adjusted her observational schedule accordingly. She also adopted other strategies, including placing herself "on-call," asking the staff to contact her at any time when a decision was about to be made so that she could be present. In practice, however, she found that the staff tended to contact her after the decision had been made. To compensate for the missing data, Anspach attempted to carry out informal interviews with at least two people who had been present when the life-and-death decision had been made. She was fully aware of the limitations of such data insofar as they had been "transformed by the memory and perceptions of my informants" (ibid.:193). Nevertheless, given the constraints under which Anspach was operating, they offered some opportunity to compare and contrast the decision-making processes that Anspach was able to observe with reports of those that had been inaccessible to her. Any differences between the interview data and the observational data would have raised questions about the generalizability of her observational findings to the cases that she had not been able to observe. These are questions that could not, of course, be answered from the interview data alone. Such data would not be able to resolve the ambiguity about whether the differences arose from the selective memory and perceptions of informants or systematic differences between the events that had been observed and those that had not. Thus while concordance between the interview data and observational data would strengthen our confidence in the generalizability of the observational findings, differences could only be resolved by further observational work. In either case, the use of multiple methods plays an important role in the search for contradictory evidence, which, as we have seen, is central to rigorous qualitative research.

Anspach's study illustrates a further way in which multiple methods can be used within a single study. On the basis of her observations, she came to the tentative conclusion that there were patterned, systematic differences between nurses and physicians in their approaches to difficult life-and-death decisions. Rather than relying upon "impressions based on observations and informant interviews," Anspach decided to test out her conclusion by conducting a series of semistructured, in-depth interviews with fellows, housestaff, and nurses in the units she observed. These interviews elicited informants' views about decision-making in relation to seven actual patients in each nursery, using prepared case histories where the staff had not been closely involved with the particular baby. Among the goals Anspach identifies for these interviews, two are relevant to our concern with providing evidence of the trustworthiness of research findings. The first was "to draw more thorough conclusions about the perceptions of staff than could be obtained by observations and informant interviews" (ibid.:219). The second was "to pursue theoretical leads and hypotheses that were suggested in the course of observations" (ibid.).

While Anspach's interviews were carried out with members of the settings in which her observations were carried out, the use of multiple methods to increase the comprehensiveness of findings can also be extended to other contexts. This is illustrated by Carolyn Wiener's (2000) participant observation study of quality assessment and improvement work in U.S. hospitals, which was discussed in Chapter 3. Toward the end of the study, when she was already beginning to write up her findings, Wiener discovered an online network where quality professionals discussed common problems and sought assistance from one another. She subscribed to the network and then made use of the twenty-five to fifty messages per day to check the universality of the issues and dilemmas she identified through her observational study and to give additional insights into how regulation and policy were negotiated in other U.S. hospital settings.

Edgerton's (1967) study of how noninstitutionalized mentally retarded people live their lives, which was discussed above, is another example of how combining different methods can strengthen our confidence in the findings from a research study. As is often the case in health research, Edgerton was interested in a phenomenon that lacked a discrete geographical location in which to carry out observational research. By definition, the ex-patients whose lives were the focus of the study were widely dispersed so they could not be observed *in situ*. Consequently, interviewing was the most practical method of data collection: as we have seen, Edgerton carried out repeated interviews with forty-eight ex-patients. Some of the problems associated with the interpretation of interview data were discussed in Chapter 5. Given Edgerton's central finding that one of the major challenges facing the ex-patients he studied was maintaining "a cloak of competence" through the careful presentation of self, total reliance on interview data would raise questions about the conclusions that might safely be drawn. However, our confidence in his conclusions is strengthened by the combination of these interviews with other sources of data. Edgerton describes how he went about this:

> Conjointly with these friendly and informal interviews, as much participant-observation as possible in the lives of the former patients was undertaken. This included trips to recreational areas, grocery shopping, shopping excursions in department stores, sight-seeing drives, social visits in their homes, invitations to restaurants, participation in housework, financial planning, parties, and visits to the homes of friends and relatives. (ibid.:17)

These examples illustrate how combining different methods of data collection within a single study can increase our confidence in the soundness of the conclusions drawn. The use of multiple methods encourages us to pay attention to the way in which particular research findings are always and inevitably the product of the circumstances in which they are produced. It may, in particular, highlight differences in the kinds of account that are produced in different contexts. Where data from two methods yield different results, the researcher can consider how such differences have arisen, offering an opportunity to refine and enrich the analysis (Jick 1979). As Hammersley and Atkinson (1995) suggest, such differences between different data sources can be just as important as similarities. Investigating discrepancies between the data generated by different methods is one more way in which the sophistication of our understanding of a particular phenomenon can be enhanced (Bryman 1988).

The use of multiple methods within a single study is sometimes termed "triangulation" (Denzin 1970; LeCompte & Goetz 1982; Lincoln & Guba

1985). The concept of triangulation is drawn from military, navigational or surveying contexts (Jick 1979; Flick 1992; Hammersley & Atkinson 1995; Nolan & Behi 1995; Janesick 1994). Hammersley and Atkinson describe how triangulation is performed in surveying:

> For someone wanting to locate their position on a map, a single landmark can only provide the information that they are situated somewhere along a line in a particular direction from that landmark. With two landmarks, however, one's exact position can be pinpointed by taking bearings on both; one is at the point on the map where the two lines cross. (1995:231)

We have steered clear of the term "triangulation" in our discussion of multiple methods in order to avoid the ambiguity with which it is sometimes associated. Triangulation is used in two subtly but significantly different ways. The first of these is akin to the use of multiple methods as discussed above, with the emphasis upon overcoming the partiality of data drawn from a single source (Silverman 1993) and increasing the comprehensiveness of a study (Oiler Boyd 1993a). The second refers to the use of multiple data sources to test the validity of findings from one of the methods used. This is the original sense of the concept as employed by Campbell and Fiske:

> Once a proposition has been confirmed by two or more independent measurement processes, the uncertainty of its interpretation is greatly reduced. ... If a proposition can survive the onslaught of a series of imperfect measures, with their irrelevant error, confidence should be placed in it. (1959:35)

The emphasis is upon counterbalancing the distorting effects of any single method with the aim of establishing the convergent validity of findings drawn from complementary approaches. Bloor summarizes this second interpretation of the term triangulation as follows: "Findings may be judged valid when different and contrasting methods of data collection yield identical results on the same research subjects" (1997:38).

There are some very significant problems with this second use of triangulation. The notion that triangulation represents a test of validity rests upon the assumption that the weaknesses of one method can be compensated for by the strengths of another. This, in turn, relies on the further assumption that different methods do not share the same weaknesses (Jick 1979). However, simply because the findings obtained from two different data sources are identical is no guarantee that they are true. It is quite possible that both are incorrect as a result of either systematic or random error (Hammersley & Atkinson 1995).

Bloor (1997) identified two particular difficulties that confront the claim that triangulation can be used to test the validity of findings. The first of these is that if we assume that given a particular research topic, there will be one best method of investigation, triangulation will necessarily involve juxtaposing findings from a superior method with those from an inferior one. This does not create difficulties so long as the findings from the two methods converge. But what are we to do if they diverge? Are we to set aside the findings from the superior method because they have not been supported by the inferior? Or would we conclude that the difference between the two sets of findings arose from a shortcoming of the inferior method? There are real logical difficulties in posing as a test of validity a technique that can be used only to corroborate findings and never to refute them (see also Trend 1979).

The second problem, raised by Bloor, concerns the practical difficulties that arise when we attempt to compare data collected using different methods. To demonstrate these difficulties, he cites his own study of death certification practices (Bloor 1994). In this study, Bloor combined in-depth interviews with clinicians with an exercise in which the same clinicians were asked to complete dummy death certificates on the basis of detailed case summaries that he provided. Bloor found that, in the interviews, clinicians described their practices in very general terms, whereas the dummy certification exercises required them to deal with very specific instances. While the data collected using the two different methods were superficially similar, he could not be sure that this was not an artifact of the lack of specificity in the interviews compared with the dummy cases. Similarly, where there were discrepancies, these could be explained by the defeasibility of the general rules offered in the interviews, the extent to which the rules could always be qualified and elaborated to fit particular circumstances. Jick made a similar point when he argued that "it is a delicate exercise to decide whether or not results have converged" (1979:607).

While, as we have just seen, there are very significant difficulties in using triangulation as a test of validity, this does not discredit the usefulness of multimethod approaches in increasing both the comprehensiveness and the credibility of findings from a research study. Where methods are chosen on sound theoretical and practical grounds, rather than the use of multiple methods being seen as an inherent good, they may add to the comprehensiveness of a study and stimulate reflexive analysis (see below) of data from different sources in relation to the circumstances of their production. As with other means of reducing the likelihood of error in qualitative research, the decision about whether to use one or more methods will often be guided by resource constraints (Bryman 1988; Jick 1979; Dootson 1995). In the next section we turn to a related technique, which, like triangulation, is sometimes (in our view, mistakenly) advocated as a test of the validity of qualitative research findings.

CHECKING RESEARCH FINDINGS
WITH RESEARCH PARTICIPANTS

A number of authors recommend the use of a practice variously known as respondent validation, host recognition, or member checking as a means of verifying the findings of qualitative research studies (Frake 1964; Lincoln & Guba 1985; Guba 1981; Sandelowski 1986; Walker 1989). Most frequently, this practice involves feeding back research findings to study participants and inviting them to comment on the adequacy of the researcher's interpretations and conclusions.

Sometimes these attempts at member checking are reserved until the end of the study. For example, in his study of surgical mistakes, Bosk (1979) waited until he had completed his report and then invited the surgeons to give their opinion of it. Others seek to elicit participant responses to their emerging analyses in the course of the data collection itself. Anspach (1993) adopted this latter approach in her study of intensive care nurseries. She describes how and why she did so:

> I occasionally shared my observations and interpretations with those I knew fairly well and solicited their opinions. I consciously reached this decision on the basis of both methodological considerations and assumptions about field relationships. Using research subjects to comment on the researcher's interpretations can yield valuable information obtainable through no other means. Direct questions enable the researcher to explore subjects' perceptions and to clarify points that remain ambiguous. These questions also serve as a validity check to determine whether professionals' accounts of their motivations, criteria, and actions are consistent with the researcher's observations and interpretations. They provide a test of what Schutz called "subjective adequacy," which may lead the researcher to revise inferences and interpretations in the light of what has been learned. (ibid.:202)

When used in this way, member checking overlaps with the use of multiple methods, which was discussed in the previous section. The researcher elicits informant understandings to compare and contrast with her own interpretations. This kind of member checking can serve a valuable purpose when it exposes the researcher to alternative interpretations of the data. When inconsistencies between the researchers' interpretations and those offered by the members of the setting are uncovered, this can stimulate researchers to reconsider taken-for-granted assumptions and revisit their preliminary conclusions. As such, member checking can help to reduce error. It offers an additional source of data, which, particularly when it is at odds with the researcher's own interpretation, can stimulate a reworking of the analysis.

However, Anspach also refers to this checking her interpretations of her data with participants as a "validity check." This idea that member checking can be seen as a test of validity is widely represented in the literature on qualitative methods. For example, Guba (1981) argued the ultimate test of validity lies in isomorphism between a study's findings and respondents' perceptions. Writing with Lincoln, nearly a decade later, he described member checks as "the single most crucial technique for establishing credibility" (Guba & Lincoln 1989:239). Among the functions that Guba and Lincoln identified for such member checks were the opportunity for assessing the intent behind a given action, for correcting errors of fact and interpretation, for obtaining additional information, for putting the respondent on record as having agreed that the researcher "got it right," for summarizing the findings, and for judging the overall adequacy of a study.

To illustrate the potential of such member checks, Guba and Lincoln took, as an example, a study that had been carried out by Skrtic and his coworkers (including Guba; Skrtic, Guba, & Knowlton 1985). Member checking was used but failed to turn up a single suggestion for correction of interpretation. Guba and Lincoln interpret this absence of dissent as indicating that "no person, no matter how powerful or remote from power, at any site, felt that her or his construction had been misrepresented" (1989:240). This, of course, is only one possible interpretation of the absence of disagreement from research participants. Alternatively, failure to uncover alternative interpretations could be taken as evidence of the insensitivity of member checking as a test of validity.

As with triangulation, there are a number of problems with the use of member checking as a test of validity. The first is suggested by Guba's expectation of isomorphism between participant and researcher accounts of phenomena. As both Bloor (1983) and Emerson and Pollner (1988) have argued, the accounts of researchers and participants are formulated in the light of very different purposes and can be expected to vary from one another in ways that are unrelated to their validity. This means that the most that such member checks can be expected to do is to ask participants to comment on whether a research account represents a "legitimate elaboration and systematization of the member's account" (Bloor 1983:157).

Even leaving aside this limitation, there are significant practical problems in using of member checking to assess the validity of research findings. Bloor (1997) cites two of his own studies, in which he made use of different forms of member checking, to illustrate some of these problems (Bloor 1976; Bloor, McKeganey, & Fonker 1988). In the first, Bloor studied regional variations in adenotonsillectomies. He observed outpatient clinics in each region, so as to be able to compare the surgical assessment practices and determine whether the variation in surgery rates could be explained by surgeons' different decision-making criteria. Bloor produced written summaries of his findings, which he then fed back to the surgeons he had observed. He interviewed the surgeons to discover whether they endorsed his analysis of the decision-making criteria that they employed. In the second study, Bloor and his colleagues carried out observations in a psychiatric day hospital (Bloor et al. 1988). Their particular focus was on informal patient culture and the hospital's group therapy program. The researchers again shared a written summary of their analysis with the professionals and the patients in the setting. This was followed by group discussions, one with patients and the other with the staff. These discussions focused upon reactions to the draft report. In a similar exercise, Emerson and Pollner (1988) took the findings from a study of psychiatric emergencies in California back to the providers of those services.

Both Bloor (1983, 1997) and Emerson and Pollner (1988) reported significant difficulties in eliciting responses to their reports from those they had studied. Taken together, these cast substantial doubt on the feasibility of using such methods as a test of validity. First, they concluded that research participants could not be relied upon to have read the reports with sufficient attention or the appropriate critical spirit for member checking to be effective. Emerson and Pollner termed this the problem of "textual reference." In the course of the member-checking exercise they were both criticized and praised by participants for things they had not in fact written. While the focus of the research and details of research findings may be of considerable interest to the researcher, there cannot be any guarantee that research participants will share this enthusiasm.

The second problem with member checks is the difficulty of disentangling participants' appraisals of the research report from their situated behavior in the context of the validation interviews. This is a special case of the problems with treating interviews as a source of objective data, which we identified in Chapter 5. For example, in the adenotonsillectomy study, Bloor found that a surgeon who initially said that he could find nothing to disagree with in the report was able, with persistent questioning, to identify several aspects that he felt were debatable. There are at least two possible interpretations of this shift. On the one hand, the surgeon may have felt reluctant to criticize Bloor's work and therefore only prepared to reveal his reservations once Bloor demonstrated through his persistence that this was expected. On the other hand, the surgeon may indeed have found little or nothing to disagree with in the report but have been led by Bloor's persistence to conclude that the research required him to identify something, anything, that was inaccurate about the report. The problem with the use of member checks as a validation exercise is that it is impossible to separate out the doctor's "true" feelings about the report from the "transactional context" (Emerson & Pollner 1988) in which they are expressed. The way in which the researcher frames his questions and probes participants' responses may tacitly direct or prestructure the responses elicited. In effect, member checking becomes a special case of the general problems of interviewing that were reviewed in Chapter 5.

The third problem with member checks as a test of validity was referred to by Emerson and Pollner as that of the "relational context." Emerson and Pollner noted that the responses to their report by at least one of their participants could be understood as an attempt to "do friendship" with the researcher. Bloor also noted that the interviews and discussions he set up were marked by what he described as consensus-seeking behavior, both by himself and by the participants. Member checks are governed by the same rules of polite behavior and etiquette as other social encounters (Bloor 1997). The concern to avoid contentious issues and to resolve any potential conflicts again complicates any attempt to use member checks as a test of validity.

A fourth problem identified by both Bloor and Emerson and Pollner is that one cannot assume that participants act as unbiased assessors when invited to comment on draft reports. As members of the setting studied, one would expect them to have their own micropolitical agenda, which would affect their evaluations. This is what Emerson and Pollner referred to as the "organizational context" of member checks.

Whereas, in the adenotonsillectomy study, Bloor carried out separate interviews with each surgeon, in the psychiatric day hospital study, he used group interviews to elicit responses to his findings. This was intended to reduce Bloor's own influence upon the interactions and the data obtained. In the event, he found that, in the absence of a strong lead from the researcher, one member of each of the discussion groups acted as chair and constrained the context in much the same way as Bloor had in the previous study. The group interviews threw up additional problems of interpretation insofar as there was disagreement among the members of the discussion groups. Some members endorsed his findings while others rejected them.

As these three studies (Bloor 1976; Bloor et al. 1988; Emerson & Pollner 1988) demonstrate, member checks cannot be treated as unproblematic tests of validity. Responses to researcher reports by participants are not "immaculately produced, but rather are shaped and constrained by the circumstances of their production" (Bloor 1983:171). This does not mean that they have no value in enhancing the trustworthiness of research. We must simply be more modest in our evaluation of their potential. Their primary contribution is in providing additional data which may cause the researcher to rethink preliminary analyses. Ironically, perhaps, the most significant contribution to error reduction that can be made by member checks does not arise when members endorse the researcher's findings and interpretations. Such endorsements bear an indeterminate relationship to the accuracy or otherwise of the analysis. Member checks are most effective when they challenge the researcher's conclusions. It is then that they fulfill the function of searching for contradictory evidence, which is central to the scientific endeavor.

FAIR DEALING

In Chapter 1, we argued that any account of a phenomenon was irreducibly an account from a particular point of view. This means that a range of different representations of the same phenomenon, which are all potentially both legitimate and true, are possible. This has important implications for researchers' truth claims and for judgments of the trustworthiness of research reports. A significant source of error in qualitative reporting lies in the practice of presenting the perspective of one individual or group as if it defines the objective truth about the phenomenon of interest, while paying scant attention to the potentially contradictory voices of alternative perspectives. We can have much greater confidence in a research report that deals even-handedly with the perspectives of all of those who are part of the setting or group studied (Dingwall 1992).

We are concerned here with the issue of partisanship in research, which has been much debated in the literature on social science research methods. In an early contribution to this debate, Howard Becker argued that research is always morally and politically partisan. The notion that it could be otherwise, he suggests, is a dangerous self-delusion that encourages us to claim that our research has identified objective reality when its subjectivity is simply camouflaged (Becker 1967). Becker's conclusion is, "The question is not whether we should take sides, since we inevitably will, but rather whose side are we on?" (ibid.:239). This call for partisanship in research is reflected in some of the arguments we discussed in Chapter 1 about the proper purposes of research. There we saw that some writers and researchers argue that the goal of research should not be the production of knowledge but rather the emancipation of oppressed groups from sources of domination. If we accept this argument, then there can be no argument against the selective presentation of perspectives and understandings of the situation to further the interests of a particular group or groups.

This is the position that Diamond (1992) adopted in his study of nursing home care, which was discussed in Chapter 8. Diamond expresses the aim underlying his research project as follows:

> I began to wonder how nursing homes operate as industrial enterprises. How does the work of caretaking become defined and get reproduced day in and

day out as a business? What is the process by which goods and services are bought and sold in this context? How, in other words, does the everyday world of Ian and Aileen [two nursing assistants known personally to Diamond] and their co-workers, and the people they tend, get turned into a system in which gray [older frail people] can get written about in financial journals as producing gold, a classic metaphor for money? What is the process of making gray gold? (ibid.:5)

It is clear from this short excerpt that Diamond interprets the provision of nursing home care as a highly exploitative process. The exploited groups are identified as nursing assistants, on the one hand, and patients on the other. Throughout the book we are given detailed, vivid, and highly sympathetic accounts of the conditions of their lives and their sometimes brutal and consistently heartless treatment within the treatment facilities where they work and live. The agents of this exploitation are, as in this excerpt, generally implied rather than identified. They are the owners and administrators of the care homes who are represented as responsible for the marketization and commodification of the care of frail elderly patients and the exploitation of the nursing assistants who carry out most of this care. Somewhat strangely, given the book's avowed aim of examining how the everyday world of the care assistants and patients is turned into an industrial enterprise, there is almost no direct attention paid to the "everyday world" of the owners and managers, who are apparently the agents of this transformation. For the most part, these actors remain shadowy, almost malign forces, on the edge of Diamond's analysis, whose behaviors and perspectives are never fully described, far less analyzed, but whose alleged greed and inhumanity serve as implicit explanations for the distressing conditions that Diamond details.

On the rare occasions when individual managers are discussed, the descriptions border on caricatures. Take, for example, the following report of an encounter between Diamond and an administrator of one of the nursing homes in which he worked:

> The administrator spotted me sipping coffee. Though we had never met, the violation caught his attention. He came up from behind me and put his arm completely around my shoulders, brought his face close to mine, and asked sarcastically, "Are you done with your coffee yet, fella? You know you could get a day of suspension for this. I just happen to be in a good mood. See that you don't do it again." He had spoken loud enough for almost everyone in the room to hear. (ibid.:50)

This anecdote about the overbearing behavior of one administrator is as close as Diamond comes to an analysis of the relations between management and staff in the homes he studied. Taking up the earlier point about searching for contradictory instances, there is no evidence of a systematic search for other such interactions to determine whether they were all characterized by the same degree of pettiness and degradation. Where administrators are discussed, the constraints under which they operate are not analyzed. They are presented as cardboard cutout characters who are "either misguided or willfully putting their own interests first" (Voysey 1975).

In commenting upon this encounter, Diamond makes clear his own commitment to partisanship:

> This too close and too loud administrator was shouting at me, whether he meant to or not, that one could take the standpoint of labor or of management, but not both, at least not simultaneously. (ibid.:51)

It is clear, then, that Diamond's lack of attention to the everyday worlds of the "villains" of his story is no accident. He has made a principled and determined decision to tell the story from the perspective of his heroes (or more accurately heroines), the predominantly black, working-class women who make up the workforce of nursing assistants in the care homes he studied.

Diamond's commitment to the perspective of the "underdog" has a long history in qualitative research. However, while the role of "champion of the underdog" may be very seductive, it raises serious questions about the confidence that can be placed in the findings of the resultant research. As Dingwall has commented elsewhere,

> Such a role undoubtedly furnishes an element of romance, radical chic even, to liven the humdrum routine of academic inquiry. It is, however, inimical to the serious practice of ethnography, whose claims to be distinguished from polemic or investigative journalism must rest on its ability to comprehend the perspectives of top dogs, bottom dogs and indeed lap dogs, and their respective contribution to the observable character of some organised social action. (1980:874)

Contrary to Becker and Diamond, we do not accept that it is either appropriate or inevitable that qualitative researchers should "take sides." In saying this, we are talking specifically about their role and activities as research scientists. It is, of course, perfectly possible that the conduct and findings of a piece of research will lead the researcher to decide that "something must be done" about a particular problem. Scientists are not required to adopt a self-denying ordinance in relation to political activism. What, in our view, they are required to do, is to make a clear distinction between their activities *qua* scientist and *qua* activist. To put it bluntly, while it is perfectly legitimate for their findings to inform their political activism, it is illegitimate for their political commitments to determine their findings.

In practice, a commitment to even-handedness and fair dealing is demonstrated when the researcher incorporates interpretations from people at all different levels of a setting or activity into the analysis. In this sense a research report should give us equal understanding of the activities of both the ostensibly powerful and the apparently powerless among those who have been studied. This is one of the characteristics that distinguishes scientific research from journalism.

Bosk's (1979) study of the management of medical mistakes is again an excellent example of a commitment to fair dealing. The surgical services that Bosk studied were characteristically hierarchical and the attending surgeons did not hesitate to wield their power in ways that can easily be interpreted as autocratic and oppressive. In his turn, Bosk does not shrink from portraying this exercise of power. For example, he reports the following incident in which one of the attending surgeons launches a vitriolic verbal attack on one of his juniors:

> On rounds, Dr. Arthur was examining the incision of Mrs. Anders, a young woman who had just received her second mastectomy. After reassuring her that everything was fine, everyone left her room. We walked a bit down the hall and Arthur exploded: "That wound looks like a piece of walking dogshit. We don't close wounds with continuous suture on this service. ... These are the fine points that separate good surgeons from butchers. ... I never want to see another wound closed like that. Never!" (ibid.:62–63)

Bosk makes it clear that the suturing that occasioned this outburst would have been perfectly acceptable on the other surgical services within the same hospital. What is at issue here is not a junior surgeon having transgressed against a professional consensus. Indeed, on another surgical service, the junior might well have been sanctioned for failing to use a continuous suture. Bosk points out the nature of the relationship between Arthur and his subordinates:

> Dr. Arthur has numerous personal eccentricities which he expects housestaff to respect and learn from. ... Given the autocratic nature of surgical authority, the strong personal preferences of superiors are translated into absolute rules of conduct for subordinates. In everyday life, we label those with this power prima donnas; their own likes and dislikes become the rules others follow. (ibid.:65)

Bosk's treatment of the senior surgical staff he observed could certainly not be described as sycophantic. He paints them "warts and all." However, they are never reduced to the status of cardboard cutout villains. His analysis allows us to understand not only the lived realities of the underdogs in the surgical hierarchy (the medical students and junior doctors) but also that of the "top dogs" (the attending surgeons). However regrettable some aspects of the attending surgeons' behavior may appear, Bosk does not simply dismiss them as irrational, malevolent, or random acts. Rather, he seeks to understand them from within their own frame of reference. It is clear that taking this stance did not come naturally to Bosk and that it involved considerable intellectual self-discipline. He describes the way in which his own structural position encouraged him to abandon fair dealing in favor of partisanship:

> There was, of course, the danger that I would identify with the structural position of being a houseofficer, even if I avoided strong attachments to specific individuals. After all, I was a twenty-four-year-old graduate student, subordinate to a dissertation committee, and struggling to achieve autonomy within my own profession. Surely there was a clear and ever-present danger that, being a subordinate myself, I would overidentify with the subordinate and his problems. ... Of course, I also had to guard against the opposite problem, overidentification with attendings. After all, did they not have, to an exaggerated degree, the autonomy I was working so hard to obtain? (ibid.:204–5)

Bosk outlines some of the practical measures that helped him to resist these temptations and achieve the fair dealing that is evident in his report. First, conversations with his wife, whose job involved supervising trainees in another health care setting, alerted him to some of the problems that superordinates face in balancing patient and subordinate needs. Second, Bosk's supervisor challenged him to analyze his data as examples of generic problems of superordinate-subordinate relations, rather than becoming enmeshed in the "specific perturbations of housestaff-attending relations" (ibid.:205). The result of Bosk's efforts is that we have a complex analysis of not only the attending surgeons' behavior as experienced by the junior staff, but also of the professional, practical, and ideological factors that hold such behavior in place.

Bosk's insightful comments on his experience of fieldwork lead us to the next means by which researchers can increase the reader's confidence in the findings of a research project—the practice of reflexivity.

REFLEXIVITY

Unrecognized reactivity is a significant threat to the validity of qualitative research findings. Reactivity is, of course, a concern for researchers in all research traditions. However, the ways in which this problem is managed vary between these different approaches. In quantitative research, the primary emphasis is upon standardizing procedures to ensure that any variability in the findings cannot be attributed to variations in data collection practices. As we have seen, qualitative researchers tend to be less convinced about the feasibility of achieving such standardization. They argue that, while it may be possible to standardize the stimulus (e.g., the wording and administration of a survey question), it is less possible to ensure that the stimulus is received, understood, and interpreted in a standardized manner. Qualitative researchers accept that the social context in which data are collected always has an impact upon those data. As Hammersley and Atkinson note, "There is no way in which we can escape the social world in order to study it" (1995:17). The presence and activities of the researcher become part of that social world and can therefore be expected to influence the data obtained. Rather than attempting the impossible task of eliminating this influence, qualitative researchers are more likely to attempt to take account of it in their data analysis. Qualitative research calls for a level of self-conscious reflection upon the ways in which the findings of research are inevitably shaped by the research process itself and for an analysis that takes this into account. By reflexivity we mean sensitivity to the way in which the researcher's presence has contributed to the data collected (whether it is interview or observational data) and how his or her assumptions have shaped the data analysis. Evidence of such reflexivity increases our confidence in the findings from such research.

The researcher's personal characteristics can be expected to have a considerable impact upon the data. In recent years, particular attention has been paid to the influence of the researcher's gender on the data obtained in interviews and fieldwork. Informants have been found to say different things to male and female researchers and access to settings or certain kinds of information within that setting are also related to gender (Becker 1967; Warren 1988). In addition, as Silverman (1993) and McKeganey and Bloor (1991) have argued, other variables such as age and occupational class may also have a significant impact on the data obtained in research settings. In the context of this book, it is important to note that, where the researcher is known to be a health professional, it is likely that the information that is given will reflect that which is deemed to be appropriate to give to a health professional. Such information is not necessarily better or worse than that which will be given to non–health professionals but it can be expected to be systematically different. Once again, it is not the data per se that are the mark of high-quality research, but the reflexivity with which they are handled and interpreted.

Reflexivity involves seeing research participants as purposively engaged in producing the activities we observe and the talk to which we listen. It requires the researcher to consider possible reasons why our research participants behave as they do in the context of our research. For example,

Edgerton (1967) was aware that the talk of ex-patients of a large state institution for the mentally retarded was highly constrained by the anxiety that they might be reinstitutionalized. For this, and other reasons, Edgerton was sensitive to the dangers of treating his informants' talk as a reproduction of what they "really think" about themselves. He incorporates this awareness into the interpretation of his data, warning the reader of the dangers of too readily accepting the informants' statements as simply "factual." For example, having presented extensive evidence that most informants maintain that they are not mentally retarded and that their confinement in the state institution was based on a wrong diagnosis and that their current difficulties are a consequence of institutionalization rather than its cause, he comments,

> By attributing their relative incompetence to the depriving experience of institutionalization, and by insisting that the institutionalization itself was unjustified, the ex-patients have available an excuse that can and does sustain self-esteem in the face of constant challenge. To what extent they "really," in any psychodynamic sense, accept their own denial is exceedingly difficult to estimate. They usually give the impression of being successful in their efforts to answer questions about themselves, but at the same time they give indication that, fundamentally, they either know or strongly suspect that they are mentally retarded. (ibid.:170)

Reflexivity also demands self-consciousness about the intellectual and personal baggage the researcher brings to the interpretation of the data. We touched on this point in our discussion of the importance of paying attention to negative evidence earlier in this chapter. As we argued there, the exposure of the data and the researcher's interpretations of that data to critical audiences, including the research participants themselves, is likely to increase sensitivity to aspects of the evidence-base that might otherwise go unremarked.

There are various measures that researchers can adopt to foster their own capacity for reflexivity. For example, keeping a field diary provides an opportunity to engage in regular self-conscious reflection upon one's impact upon the settings and participants studied. When it comes to analyzing the data, the entries in such field diaries can be an invaluable aid to interpretation of the data recorded in the field notes. Similarly, taking regular "time out" from the fieldwork can help to foster a reflexive attitude, as we saw earlier in relation to Bosk's (1979) study of the management of surgical mistakes. Third, regular discussions with research mentors and supervisors can encourage one to achieve the kind of distance from the research process that is fundamental to reflexivity. In assessing the likelihood of error in research findings, the research consumer can look for evidence of the kind of self-conscious monitoring that these various practices represent.

Various means of assessing the researcher's impact upon the data obtained have also been proposed. These include comparing statements that are made to the researcher alone, and those made in the presence of others (Silverman 1989). Reflection on how the data obtained have changed over time can be illuminating. For example, in their analysis of humor in an outpatient clinic, Yoels and Clair (1995) chart changes in the way in which doctors and nurses in the setting joked with the researchers themselves over the two years in which they carried out the fieldwork. They interpret these changes as an indicator of their changing relationship with the members of the setting they studied:

> In looking at the responses of newcomers [i.e., the researchers] to the setting over time, we can discern important features of humor as a qualitative methodological "barometer" of outsiders' growing familiarity with, and integration into, a previously "strange" world. (ibid.:51)

Reflexivity is a matter of degree and there is no simple test to determine whether or not a researcher has achieved it to a sufficient extent. Nevertheless, consideration of how researchers have embedded their findings in an analysis of the context of their production will be an important concern in assessing the likely truth of claims that are made on the basis of those data.

Throughout this chapter, we have stressed that evaluating the evidence upon which claims derived from research are based is a responsibility that researchers and the readers and users of their reports share (Glaser & Strauss 1965a). In particular, the researcher can be expected to supply readers with the information needed to make a judgment about the likelihood that claims are true or erroneous. In our discussion of the basis on which judgments about the likely truth of findings from qualitative research are made, we now turn explicitly to the quality of the information about the process of data collection and analysis on which such judgments depend.

EXPOSITION OF PROCESS OF DATA COLLECTION AND ANALYSIS

As Athens (1984) has argued, the credibility or otherwise of a study is not something intrinsic. Rather it is something for researchers to establish in reporting their research. In coming to a judgment about the trustworthiness of findings, the reader/user needs to be able to relate the researcher's claims to the process by which he or she arrived at them. Such a judgment will take into account "the range of events the researcher saw, whom he interviewed, who talked to him, what kinds of experiences he had, and how he might have appeared to the various people whom he studied" (Glaser & Strauss 1965a:9). It also requires knowledge of the process of analysis through which the researcher derived the findings from the data obtained.

In Chapter 1, we discussed the recent vogue for abandoning conventional scientific forms of writing in favor of literary experiments. In the study of U.S. nursing homes that we discussed earlier in this chapter, Diamond reports how he adopted such an unconventional approach to writing up his research findings:

> In trying to preserve the context in which things were said and done, I employ a novel-like format so that the reading might move along as in a story. ... In pursuit of the same objective, I often choose not to pause to indicate which nursing home each speaker was in, but rather to organize comments made in different settings around the key themes they illuminate. (1992:7)

Diamond certainly succeeds in the objective he sets himself. He has produced an elegant, compelling, at times harrowing, story of the daily lives of staff and residents of the nursing homes he studied. He has challenged the inhumanity and brutality of the system in which they operate. However, his deliberate espousal of a "novel-like format" leaves us unable to make any independent judgment of the evidence upon which his story is based or to explore the possibility that the data might have been interpreted differently. Diamond, in effect, depends upon privilege of presence. His implicit claim was that he was there and so we must take his word for the authenticity of his findings. Diamond makes it clear that his primary motive for carrying out the study was political and it may well be that the format he has chosen is a more effective means of achieving his goals than a conventional scientific report. However, his approach seriously imbalances what we take to be the joint responsibility of researcher and reader to judge how convincing the evidence base for research findings actually is. In the absence of clear and explicit links between the data presented and the circumstances of their production, the reader's ability to make such judgments is significantly compromised.

As we argued in Chapter 1, the primary requirement of any scientific report is that it should lay itself open to rational assessment of its claims. Such rational assessment depends, above all, upon the provision of clear information about how the evidence on which claims are based was collected and how the conclusions were derived from that evidence. This requirement is as salient to qualitative research as to research in other traditions. It is this that allows the reader to form a judgment about the likelihood that the claims made are erroneous.

In assessing the degree of likely error in research findings, the reader is assisted by information on various aspects of how the research was carried out. The first of these concerns how access to the research setting and participants was negotiated. This can be expected to have a significant influence on the data obtained. Anspach describes, in detail, the process by which she gained access to the intensive care nursery in which she carried out most of her fieldwork. Her formal negotiation of access was, as she puts it, "deceptively simple" (1993:185). She approached the director of the nursery and the attending neonatologist with a written version of her research proposal and neither objected to what she wanted to do. They introduced her to the head nurse and the social worker, neither of whom appear to have raised any objections. Thus her initial entry to her research setting met with little resistance. However, she soon discovered that physical access to the nursery did not necessarily lead to the kind of close working relationship with nursery staff that would enable her to obtain the data on decision-making, which were the object of her study. In her own words, she often felt that she had entered a "closed society" (ibid.). These relational barriers were exacerbated by Anspach's initial unfamiliarity with the "vast knowledge of medical terminology needed to understand even the simplest interactions in the nursery" (ibid.:189). Throughout her early fieldwork, she was unable to understand much of what was said by the doctors, who spoke largely in numerical data and coded abbreviations. Anspach gives a detailed account of how her research, and the data obtained, were heavily constrained by continuous and delicate negotiations required to gain access to and understanding of the interactions that were the central focus of her study. She discusses these in terms of what she calls the "dilemma of discretion":

> Researchers frequently make decisions in which they balance the need for data and information against assumptions about field relationships, considerations of etiquette, and, in short, demands for discretion. (ibid.:195)

A strength of Anspach's work is that she not only recognizes that these decisions have an impact on the quality and comprehensiveness of the data obtained, but she also examines her data to determine the impact upon her findings. Her observations on this score are helpful to the reader who is concerned to form a judgment about the trustworthiness of the claims Anspach makes.

The discerning reader also needs detailed information about the means by which the data on which the researcher's claims are based were acquired. In particular, the reader needs to be told about how the researcher presented him- or herself, any evidence of trust or suspicion that was observed, the types of data obtained, and the length of time spent interviewing or observing. All of these factors have important implications for the quality of the data obtained. Different data collection methods will have different requirements in this regard. For example, if the main data source is interviews, the reader needs detailed information about how the interviews were carried out and, in particular, the extent to which the interview data were stimulated by direct questioning or were offered spontaneously by the informants. If, on the other hand, findings are based on observational data, the role that the observer took within the setting is an important consideration.

In judging the findings of research, the reader also needs good information about how the data were analyzed. In recent years, qualitative researchers have come under considerable criticism for their failure to clarify the process by which their findings were derived from the data and the apparent expectation that the reader should take this process on trust (Altheide & Johnson 1994; Guba & Lincoln 1989; Silverman 1989; Dingwall 1992). There have been calls for the process of data analysis to be made "semipublic and not magical" (Silverman 1989). There are at least two issues here. The first concerns the process by which the data are coded and categorized in qualitative research. The second relates to the way in which conclusions are drawn from the data obtained.

Most quantitative research methods require the researcher to clarify and operationalize the core concepts used in a study before the data are collected. In principle, at least, it is clear what can or cannot legitimately be counted as an example of a particular concept. The inductive nature of qualitative research means that the core concepts may only emerge during the course of the investigation. The clarification of concepts is often a continuous process throughout the research. The researcher develops a rudimentary classification or coding scheme on the basis of early data. This is then refined, having been exposed to further data. The most important thing is that, by the time that the study is reported, clear and unambiguous definitions of the key concepts are available.

Some researchers make use of interrater reliability checks to assess the clarity and precision of the concepts used and the consistency of their application to the data. For example, an independent panel may be supplied with the coding definitions, developed and applied to the corpus of data by the researcher(s), and asked to code a subset of the data. By calculating the level of agreement between the coding panel and the research team, it is possible to judge the explicitness of the concepts used (Hinds, Scandrett-Hibden, & McAulay 1990). Interrater reliability exercises of this kind are resource intensive and may be impractical in many studies. However, the credibility of research findings is enhanced wherever the researchers provide clear definitions of the concepts they use in their analysis. Such definitions are a public product that make the researcher's tacit assumptions explicit and allow the reader to evaluate the claims made in relation to the definitions employed (Henwood & Pidgeon 1992).

If readers are to be convinced that the researchers' claims are sound then they will need evidence that the conclusions drawn are justified in terms of the data that have been analyzed. The first requirement here is that the evidence base is trustworthy. There is a number of ways in which such trustworthiness can be enhanced. The use of mechanical recording (video or audio recording) reduces the possibility of misreporting of data, although in many circumstances these technologies may be impractical. Similarly, the use of standardized practices for the transcription of data reduces the possibility that error is introduced at this stage. In observational studies, confidence in the quality of the data will be increased when there is evidence that the researchers have spent an extended period of time in the setting that is under study.

In forming a view about the soundness of research claims, the reader also needs some means to judge the adequacy of the researchers' interpretations. A primary consideration here is the opportunity to scrutinize the data on which such interpretations are based. This requires the researcher to present substantial portions of data, whether from interviews, documents, or from observational fieldnotes, alongside the conclusions drawn. The reader can then assess whether the conclusions are justified and consider whether any possible, alternative explanations for the data could reasonably be sustained. Once again, the emphasis here is upon exposing the researcher's claims to refutation.

Throughout this chapter, we have been concerned with the basis upon which readers of research might form a judgment about the likelihood that the claims contained in a research report are justified and that the possibility of error has been limited to the greatest extent possible. This is not, of course, the only criterion that we might want to apply to the research products. Hammersley (1990) has argued convincingly that research should also be relevant "however remotely" to some public concern. It is to this issue, of the relevance of research, that we now turn.

RELEVANCE

The relationship between relevance and trustworthiness is asymmetrical. Unless claims can be trusted, they have little or no relevance to either policymakers or practitioners. On the other hand, claims can be true but irrelevant because they are trivial or insignificant. Nevertheless, as Hammersley (1990) argues, we must be wary of defining relevance in terms that are too narrow. In particular, policymakers and practitioners are not always in the best position to judge whether proposed research is or is not likely to be relevant. One of the opportunities that qualitative research, with its distinctive orientation toward discovery, offers is the possibility of providing new perspectives and developing new terms of reference, for the investigation of health care and health care settings. In doing so, it is not always helpful to take a problem as defined by policymakers and practitioners as the starting point. As Silverman argues,

> Paradoxically, by refusing to begin from a common conception of what is "wrong" in a setting, we may be most able to contribute to the identification both of what is going on and, thereby, how it may be modified in pursuit of desired ends. (1993:184–85)

This point is well illustrated by a consideration of Bosk's (1992) study of genetic counseling in a pediatric hospital, which was first discussed in Chapter 3. Unusually, as we have noted, Bosk was invited to carry out this study by the genetic counselors he eventually observed. They were conscious that theirs was a new service and, keen to provide their services as sensibly as possible, were eager to receive help from a sociologist. They were looking for research that would be highly relevant to practice. Bosk identified two outcomes that they hoped for from this collaboration. On the one hand, they were looking for a "hard-headed, objective assessment of how they were managing problems" (ibid.:6). Bosk compares this to the role of an "efficiency expert." On the other, they expected that Bosk would provide "a catalogue of the typical problems that they face but lack adequate resources to resolve" (ibid.). Here the assumption was that Bosk's findings would provide scientific support for the genetic counselors' attempts to develop their services. Bosk makes it clear that he did not interpret the counselors' expectations as cynical or self-interested. They genuinely believed in the justness of their aspirations and the benefits that they offered to clients. Once exposed to their daily reality, they anticipated that Bosk would come to share their point of view.

We can see that the definition of relevance with which the genetic counselors were operating, when they initiated the research, was somewhat limited. Bosk's own aspirations were different. He describes his approach in this way:

> Procedurally, I examine these situations to uncover what rhetoric, rationales, maxims, myths, data, and bottom lines physicians arm themselves with when they recommend one course rather than another to patients, when they explain unexpected, unwanted outcomes, and when they search for reasons to explain pain and suffering.(ibid.:4)

Echoing Silverman, the task that Bosk set himself was to identify what was "going on" in the genetic counseling service he observed. Bosk referred to this as "describing without sentimentality the way the world works" (ibid.:17). To the counselors themselves this might seem like a trivial task. They might well argue that, as people immersed in the service on a day-to-day basis, they had no need of someone else telling them what was going on. Bosk's reflection on what research like his can in fact contribute is:

> Fieldwork ... allows us to see the embedded tensions that lie beneath the surface of a rapidly advancing and dazzling medical technology: What is help? How is it provided in society at this time? ... Fieldwork allows us to describe social life as we live it.
>
> ... When it is performed with skill, it allows us to examine the shadow that falls between the image and the reality. In the case of genetic counselors, this has meant matching the counselors' statements about intent and purpose with daily encounters. (ibid.:18–19)

Bosk's findings are some way from those that the genetic counselors anticipated when they first invited him to study their service. This does not, however, render them any the less relevant. Indeed, Bosk's book stands as a testament to the potential that qualitative research has for unpacking the complexity of everyday situations. Such knowledge has a vital role to play wherever we seek to modify current practice in order to achieve some desired goal.

Originality is an important element of relevance. Unless research studies add something to our current state of knowledge their relevance is severely limited. Studies that ignore or gloss over the existing knowledge base are unlikely to make a major contribution. This is not, of course, to argue against the investigation of topics or settings that have already been studied. Rather it is to argue for the systematic building of new research upon the existing knowledge base. We have argued throughout this chapter that current knowledge is always provisional. We saw, for example, how Taylor's (2000) recent study of the Dukes family led to the modification and refinement of some of the claims from Edgerton's much earlier study of ex-residents of a state institution for people with mental retardation (Edgerton 1967). One of the strengths of Taylor's study is that it takes account of Edgerton's previous findings and is able to relate the new data to them.

The relevance of research findings is also related to the issue of their generalizability. The frequent reliance of qualitative research studies on a single case or a small number of cases raises particular difficulties in this respect. In Chapter 6, we discussed the various means by which qualitative researchers can strengthen both the empirical and the theoretical generalizability of their research findings and we shall not repeat that discussion here. Suffice it to say that, as always, it is incumbent upon researchers to provide evidence to support claims that their research findings have relevance beyond the immediate context in which they developed. Like other aspects of "goodness" in research, generalizability is a quality that has to be demonstrated rather than simply asserted or ascribed.

CONCLUSION

Throughout this chapter, we have argued that judgments about the security of research findings are never final. The hallmark of science is the pursuit of truth and the limitation of error. As such, science is an attitude of mind rather than a set of procedures. The defining characteristic of that attitude is a commitment to subject any claim to rigorous evaluation and the conscientious seeking out of evidence that might contradict or modify that claim. We have discussed some of the ways in which the findings from qualitative research may be subjected to evaluation by both researcher and the consumer of research findings. We do not put these forward as a list of requirements for the proper conduct of qualitative research studies. Rather, we offer them as examples of some of the ways in which the principle of exposing the claims of research to the systematic search for contradictory evidence might be operationalized in practice.

Envoi

This book has a simple message: qualitative methods are indispensable to the efficient, effective, fair and compassionate planning and delivery of health care. They provide rigorous descriptions of the routine, taken-for-granted practices that are so familiar as to pass unnoticed by those involved with health care organizations. When policymakers, managers or clinicians try to make changes for the benefit of patients, they need to understand these features, and the structures and contingencies that hold them in place. These aspects of health care delivery are inaccessible with quantitative techniques.

Qualitative methods also answer the "how" questions asked by managers, planners, clinicians, and users. They capture the dynamic, processual aspects of institutional life that are invisible in input-output studies. Their flexibility facilitates the discovery of the unanticipated consequences of programs and developments, consequences that would otherwise undermine their benefits. These methods identify contextual factors that either enhance or undermine the implementation of initiatives that have been shown to be beneficial under controlled conditions. They throw light on hidden aspects of health care organizations and identify the structural and interactional features that hold inappropriate behaviors in place.

This contribution has been endangered by the romantic turn in qualitative research. It is jeopardized by the enthusiasm in some circles for assimilating the social sciences to the humanities and by commitments to using research to promote ideological projects. The program that we have put forward is an unrepentantly scientific one. It is entirely possible to generate a trustworthy and relevant evidence-base for health care policy and practice through qualitative research. This possibility is founded on an alternative commitment to discipline, rigor and the subjection of one's prior assumptions to challenge and revision. While it may be impossible to establish incontrovertible truths, as some once believed, it is entirely possible to limit the range of potential error and to build a cumulative knowledge base. We insist on dealing fairly with the perspectives of members at all levels of organizations, including those whose behaviors we may find personally offensive. Indeed, examining how and why unhelpful practices are developed and sustained may be a more effective means of promoting humanity and fairness in health care organizations than celebrating the perspectives of the down-trodden and oppressed. Properly conducted, qualitative research produces findings that are sufficiently certain to justify their use to inform policy and practice.

The hallmark of all science is the rigorous search for evidence to contradict prior assumptions or hypotheses. This is, of course, the logic behind the null hypothesis in experimental studies. It is also the logic that underpins the program that we advocate here. Throughout this book, we have discussed the wide range of ways in which qualitative researchers can expose their emerging analyses to the possibility of contradiction. They must seek to identify and test alternative explanations for their observations. They must track down new observations to challenge or limit conclusions based on current knowledge. This search for negative evidence characterizes all phases of rigorous qualitative research from initial design to data analysis.

This openness to contradiction also underpins another central feature of rigorous qualitative research—the commitment to understand data in the context of their production. There is no possibility of producing data "untouched by human hands." All data have been transformed in the process of collection. They are never a pure copy of reality. Rigor demands that we subject all data, whether participants' accounts or documents or observers' records and recordings, to an analysis that relates them to the circumstances under which they were generated.

All kinds of research raise complex ethical issues in relation to the proper treatment of participants. If anything, the risks associated with quantitative research, particularly research involving experimental interventions, are more intractable than those that arise in most qualitative studies. However, it seems that IRBs currently are better equipped to deal with quantitative research designs. The criteria and rules of thumb they employ to reach their judgments are often a poor fit when applied to qualitative research. This has two adverse consequences. First, "rules," developed in the context of quantitative research, may constrain qualitative research in ways that are irrelevant and inappropriate. The cost of misdirected ethical review may be an unethical denial of benefits to commissioners and consumers. Second, and perhaps more importantly, ritualistic observation of such rules by qualitative researchers may lull IRBs into complacency, distracting them from the ethical issues that are specific to qualitative research. Qualitative researchers and IRBs need to collaborate in developing method-sensitive judgments about qualitative studies and a better understanding of the balance between risks and benefits.

The choice between qualitative and quantitative research methods should be made in relation to the question to be investigated rather than prior political, philosophical, or methodological commitments. Sometimes, the research question will be most effectively and efficiently addressed using either qualitative or quantitative methods alone. Very often, however, a combination of methods will be required to fully address the issues at hand. Sometimes, qualitative research will be the junior partner in the alliance. It may, for example, be used in the preliminary phases of a primarily quantitative study to help clarify the research question, generate hypotheses that fit and work and aid conceptualization of the key variables. Alternatively, it may be used alongside an intervention study to relate the outcome measures to the process through which they were generated, informing the interpretation of the quantitative data and enhancing the generalizability of the findings. At times, qualitative research will play the primary role, but use quantitative data to identify the problem to be examined or to inform the selection of an appropriate sample.

No single research method is exclusively capable of providing the kind of evidence base that is required to plan and deliver an effective, efficient, equitable, and humane health care system. The full range of current research technologies must be used in a flexible and informed fashion. This book has shown how qualitative research can contribute its share to this project.

References

Abrums, M. (2000). Jesus will fix it after a while: Meanings and health. *Social Science and Medicine* 50:89–105.

Adler, P. (1985). *Wheeling and Dealing: An Ethnography of an Upper-Level Drug Dealing and Smuggling Community*. New York: Columbia University Press.

Agar, M. H. (1980). *The Professional Stranger: An Informal Introduction to Ethnography*. New York: Academic Press.

Allen, D. (1997). The nursing-medical boundary: A negotiated order? *Sociology of Health and Illness* 19(4):498–520.

Altheide, D., & Johnson, J. (1994). Criteria for assessing interpretive validity in qualitative research. In N. Denzin & Y. Lincoln (Eds.), *Handbook of Qualitative Research*, 1st ed. (pp. 485–99). Thousand Oaks, CA: Sage.

Anderson, G. (1989). Critical ethnography in education: Origins, current status and new directions. *Review of Educational Research* 59(3):249–70.

Anleu, S. R. (2001). The legal regulation of medical science. *Law & Policy* 23:417–40.

Annas, G. J., & Grodin, M. A. (1992). *Nazi Doctors and the Nuremberg Code: Human Rights in Human Experiments*. Oxford: Oxford University Press.

Anspach, R. R. (1993). *Deciding Who Lives: Fateful Choices in the Intensive-Care Nursery*. Berkeley: University of California Press.

Athens, L. (1984). Scientific criteria for evaluating qualitative studies. In N. K. Denzin (Ed.), *Studies in Symbolic Interaction 5* (pp. 259-68). Greenwich, CT: JAI.

Atkinson, P. (1979). Research design in ethnography. In DE304 Course Team (Ed.), *Research Methods in Education and the Social Sciences*, (Block 3B, pp. 41–81). Milton Keynes: Open University Press.

Atkinson, P. (1990). *The Ethnographic Imagination: Textual Constructions of Reality*. London: Routledge.

Austin, D. A. (1996). Kaleidoscope: The same and different. In C. Ellis & A. Bochner (Eds.), *Composing Ethnography: Alternative Forms of Qualitative Writing* (pp. 206–30). Walnut Creek, CA: Altamira.

Bar-On, D. (1996). Ethical issues in biographical interviews and analysis. In R. Josselson (Ed.), *Ethics and Process in the Narrative Study of Lives* (pp. 9–21). Thousand Oaks, CA: Sage.

Barnes, J. (1979). *Who Should Know What? Social Science, Privacy and Ethics.* Harmondsworth: Penguin.

Baruch, G. (1981). Moral tales: Parents' stories of encounters with the health profession. *Sociology of Health and Illness* 3(3):275–96.

Baum, F. (1995). Researching public health: behind the qualitative-quantitative methodological debate. *Social Science and Medicine* 40(4):459–68.

Bayer, R. (1987). *Homosexuality and American Psychiatry.* Princeton, NJ: Princeton University Press.

Beauchamp, C. J. (1993). The c entrality of caring: A case study. In P. O. Munhall & C. Oiler Boyd (Eds.) *Nursing Research: A Qualitative Perspective,* 2nd ed. (pp. 338–58). New York: National League for Nursing.

Beauchamp, T. L., Faden, R., & Wallace, R. J., Jr. (1982). *Ethical Issues in Social Science Research.* Baltimore, MD: Johns Hopkins University Press.

Beauchamp,T. L., & Childress, J. F. (2001). *Principles of Biomedical Ethics,* 5th ed. New York: Oxford University Press.

Becker, H. S. (1967). Whose side are we on? *Social Problems* 14:239–48.

Becker, H. S. (1970). *Sociological Work: Method and Substance.* Chicago: Aldine.

Becker, H. S., & Geer, B. (1960). Participant observation: The analysis of qualitative data. In R. Adams & J. Preiss (Eds.), *Human Organization Research: Field Relations and Techniques* (pp. 267–89). Homewood, IL: Dorsey.

Becker, H. S., Geer, B., Hughes, E. C., & Strauss, A. L. (1961). *Boys in White.* Chicago: University of Chicago Press.

Beecher, H. (1959). Experimentation in man. *Journal of the American Medical Association* 169:461–78.

Beecher, H. (1966). Ethics and clinical research. *New England Journal of Medicine,* 24:1345–60.

Benatar, S. R. (1997). Just health care beyond individualism: Challenges for North American bioethics. *Cambridge Quarterly of Health Care Ethics* 6:397–415.

Billig, M., & Schegloff, E. A. (1999). Critical discourse analysis and conversation analysis: an exchange between Michael Billig and Emanuel A. Schegloff. *Discourse and Society* 10(4):543-82.

Bloor, M. (1976). Bishop Berkeley and the adenotonsillectomy enigma: An exploration of variation in the social construction of medical disposals. *Sociology* 10(1):43–61.

Bloor, M. (1983). Notes on member validation. In R. M. Emerson (Ed.), *Contemporary Field Research: A Collection of Readings* (pp. 156–72). Prospect Heights, IL: Waveland.

Bloor, M. (1994). On the conceptualisation of routine medical decision-making: Death certification as a habitual activity. In M. Bloor & P. Taraborrelli (Eds.), *Qualitative Studies in Health and Medicine* (pp. 96–109). Aldershot: Avebury.

Bloor, M. (1997). Techniques of validation in qualitative research: A critical commentary. In G. Miller & R. Dingwall (Eds.), *Context and Method in Qualitative Research* (pp. 37–50). London: Sage.

Bloor, M., McKeganey, N., & Fonker, D. (1988). *One Foot in Eden. A Sociological Study of the Range of Therapeutic Community Practice.* London: Routledge & Kegan Paul.

Bloor, M., Frankland, J., Thomas, M., & Robson, K. (2001). *Focus Groups in Social Research.* London: Sage.

Bluebond-Langer, M. (1980). *The Private Worlds of Dying Children*. Princeton, NJ: Princeton University Press.

Blumer, H. (1969). *Symbolic Interactionism*. Englewood Cliffs, NJ: Prentice Hall.

Borland, K. (1991). "That's not what I said": Interpretive conflict in oral narrative research. In S. Gluck and D. Patai (Eds.) *Women's Words: The Feminist Practice of Oral History* (pp. 63-76). New York: Routledge.

Bosk, C. L. (1979). *Forgive and Remember: Managing Medical Failure*. Chicago: University of Chicago Press.

Bosk, C. L. (1992). *All God's Mistakes: Genetic Counseling in a Pediatric Hospital*. Chicago: University of Chicago Press.

Bosk, C.L. (2000). The sociological imagination and bioethics. In Bird, C.E., Conrad, P.,& Fremont, A.M. (Eds.) *Handbook of Medical Sociology* 5th ed. (pp. 398-410). Upper Saddle River, NJ, Prentice Hall.

Bowler, I. (1995). Further notes on record taking and making in maternity care: The case of South Asian descent women. *Sociological Review* 43(1):36–51.

Britten, N. (1995). Qualitative research: Qualitative interviews in medical research. *British Medical Journal* 311:251–54.

Bryman, A. (1988). *Quantity and Quality in Social Research*. London: Unwin Hyman.

Bryman, A., & Burgess, R. G. (1994) *Analysing Qualitative Data*. London: Routledge.

Buckholdt, D., & Gubrium, J. (1979). *Caretakers: Treating Emotionally Disturbed Children*. Beverly Hills, CA: Sage.

Bulmer, M. (1980). Comment on the ethics of covert methods. *British Journal of Sociology* 31(1):59–65.

Bulmer, M. (1997). *Social Research Ethics*. London: Macmillan.

Campbell, D. (1994). Can we overcome world-view incommensurability/relativity in trying to understand the other? In R. Jessor, A. Colby, & R. Shweder (Eds.), *Ethnography and Human Development: Context and Meaning in Social Inquiry* (pp. 153–72). Chicago: University of Chicago Press.

Campbell, D., & Fiske D. (1959). Convergent and discriminant validation by multitrait multi-dimensional matrix. *Psychological Bulletin* 56:81–105.

Casper, M. J. (1998). *The Making of the Unborn Patient: Medical Work and the Politics of Reproduction in Experimental Fetal Surgery*. New Brunswick, NJ: Rutgers University Press.

Cassell, J. (1978). Risk and benefit to subjects of fieldwork, *American Sociologist* 13(3):134–43.

Cassell, J. (1979). Regulating fieldwork: Of subjects, subjection and intersubjectivity. In M. Wax & J. Cassell (Eds.), *Federal Regulations: Ethical Issues and Social Research* (pp. 129-44). Boulder, CO: Westview.

Cassell, J. (1982). Does risk-benefit analysis apply to moral evaluation of social research. In T. Beauchamp, R. Faden, R. Wallace, & L. Walters (Eds.), *Ethical Issues in Social Science Research*. Baltimore, MD: Johns Hopkins University Press.

Cassell, J., & Wax, M. (1980). Editorial introduction: Toward a moral science of human beings. *Social Problems* 27:259–64.

Castaneda, C. (1970). *The Teachings of Don Juan*. Harmondsworth: Penguin.

"Cesara, M." (1982). *Reflections of a Woman Anthropologist: No Hiding Place*. London: Academic Press.

Charmaz, K. (1995). Between positivism and postmodernism: Implications for methods. In N. K. Denzin (Ed.), *Studies in Symbolic Interaction 17* (pp. 43–72). Greenwich, CT: JAI.

Christians, C. G. (2000). Ethics and politics in qualitative research. In N. K. Denzin & Y. Lincoln (Eds.), *Handbook of Qualitative Research*, 2nd ed. (pp. 133–55). Thousand Oaks, CA: Sage.

Church, J.T. (2002) For the record: Should all disciplines be subject to the Common Rule? Human subjects of social science research. *Academe* 88(3): http://www.aaup.org/publications/Academe/02mj/02mjftr.htm

Cicourel, A. V. (1964). *Method and Measurement in Sociology.* New York: Free Press.

Clifford, J. (1981). On ethnographic surrealism. *Comparative Studies in Society and History* 23(4):539–64.

Clifford, J. (1986). Partial truths. In J. Clifford & G. E. Marcus (Eds.), *Writing Culture: The Poetics and Politics of Ethnography* (pp. 1–26). Berkeley: University of California Press.

Cochrane, A. L. (1972). *Effectiveness and Efficiency: Random Reflections on Health Services.* London: Nuffield Provincial Hospitals Trust.

Cornwell, J. (1984). *Hard-Earned Lives: Accounts of Health and Illness from East London.* London: Tavistock.

Crabtree, B. F., & Miller, W. L. (1991). A qualitative approach to primary care research: The long interview. *Family Medicine* 23(2):145–51.

Davis, F. (1963). *Passage through Crisis: Polio Victims and Their Families.* Indianapolis: Bobbs Merrill.

Davis, K. (1988). *Power under the Microscope.* Dordrecht: Foris.

Dawson, L. L., & Prus, R. (1995). Postmodernism and linguistic reality vs. symbolic interactionism and obdurate reality. In N. Denzin (Ed.), *Studies in Symbolic Interaction 17* (pp. 105–24). Greenwich CT: JAI.

de Vries, H., Weijts, W., Dijkstra, M., & Kok, G. (1992). The utilization of qualitative and quantitative data for health education program planning, implementation and evaluation: A spiral approach. *Health Education Quarterly* 19(1):101–15.

De Mille, R. (1976). *Castaneda's Journey: The Power and the Allegory.* Santa Barbara, CA: Capra.

De Mille, R. (Ed.) (1980) *The Don Juan Papers: Further Castaneda Controversies.* Santa Barbara, CA: Ross-Erickson.

Denscombe, M. (1983). Interviews, accounts and ethnographic research on teachers. In M. Hammersley (Ed.), *The Ethnography of Schooling* (pp. 107-28). Driffield: Nafferton.

Denzin, N. (1970). *The Research Act in Sociology.* London: Butterworth.

Denzin, N. (1971). The logic of naturalistic inquiry. *Social Forces* 50:166–82.

Denzin, N. (1983). Interpretive interactionism. In G. Morgan (Ed.), *Beyond Method: Strategies for Social Research* (pp. 129-46). Beverly Hills, CA: Sage.

Denzin, N., & Lincoln, Y. (1994). Entering the field of qualitative research. In N. Denzin & Y. Lincoln (Eds.), *Handbook of Qualitative Research*, 1st ed. (pp. 1–17). Thousand Oaks, CA: Sage.

Denzin, N., & Lincoln, Y. (2000). *Handbook of Qualitative Research*, 2nd ed. Thousand Oaks, CA: Sage.

Dewey, J. (1938). *Logic: The Theory of Inquiry.* New York: Henry Holt.

Diamond, T. (1992). *Making Gray Gold*. Chicago: University of Chicago Press.

DiMaggio, P. J., & Powell, W.W. (1983). The iron cage revisited: Institutional isomorphism and collective rationality in organizational fields. *American Sociological Review* 48 (2):147-60.

Dingwall, R. (1977). *The Social Organisation of Health Visitor Training*. London: Croom Helm.

Dingwall, R. (1980). Ethics and ethnography. *Sociological Review* 28(4):871–91.

Dingwall, R. (1992). Don't mind him he's from Barcelona: Qualitative methods in health studies. In J. Daly, I. McDonald, & E. Willis (Eds.), *Researching Health Care* (pp. 161–75). London: Tavistock/Routledge.

Dingwall, R. (1997). Accounts, interviews and observations. In G. Miller & R. Dingwall (Eds.), *Context and Method in Qualitative Research* (pp. 51–65). London: Sage.

Dingwall, R. (2001). *Aspects of Illness*. Aldershot: Ashgate.

Dingwall, R., & Murray, T. (1983). Categorisation in accident departments: "Good" patients, "bad" patients and "children." *Sociology of Health and Illness* 5(2): 127–48.

Dingwall, R. and Strong, P. M. (1985). The interactional study of organizations: A critique and reformulation. *Urban Life* 14:205–31.

Dingwall, R., Eekelaar, J. M., & Murray, T. (1983). *The Protection of Children: State Intervention and Family Life*. Oxford: Basil Blackwell.

Dingwall, R., Tanaka, H., & Minamikata, S. (1991). Images of parenthood in the United Kingdom and Japan. *Sociology* 25:423–46.

Dingwall, R., Murphy, E., Watson, P., Greatbatch D., & Parker, S. (1998). Catching goldfish: Quality in qualitative research, *Journal of Health Services Research and Policy* 3:167–72.

Dodier, N., & Camus, A. (1998). Openness and specialization: dealing with patients in a hospital emergency service. *Sociology of Health and Illness* 20:413–44.

Dootson, S. (1995). An in-depth study of triangulation. *Journal of Advanced Nursing* 22(1):183–87.

Douglas, M., & Nicod M. (1974). Taking the biscuit: The structure of British meals. *New Society* (19 December):744–47.

Dowling, A. F., Jr. (2001). Do hospital staff interfere with computer system implementation? *Health Care Management Review* 5:3–32.

Duffy, M. E. (1987). Methodological triangulation: A vehicle for merging quantitative and qualitative research methods. *Image: Journal of Nursing Scholarship* 19(3):130–33.

Edgerton, R. B. (1967). *The Cloak of Competence*. Berkeley: University of California Press.

Eisner, E. (1983). Anastasia might still be alive, but the monarchy is dead. *Educational Researcher* 12(5):13-14.

Ellis, C. (1995). Emotional and ethical quagmires in returning to the field. *Journal of Contemporary Ethnography* 24(1):68–98.

Ellis, C. (1996). Maternal connections. In C. Ellis & A. Bochner (Eds.), *Composing Ethnography: Alternative Forms of Qualitative Writing* (pp. 240–43). Walnut Creek, CA: Altamira.

Ellis, C., & Bochner, A. (1992). Telling and performing personal stories: The constraints of choice in abortion. In C. Ellis & M. Flaherty (Eds.), *Investigating Subjectivity: Research on Lived Experience* (pp. 79–101). Newbury Park, CA: Sage.

Ellis, C., & Bochner, A. (Eds.) (1996). *Composing Ethnography: Alternative Forms of
Qualitative Writing.* Walnut Creek, CA: Altamira.

Ellis, C., & Flaherty, M. (1992). *An Agenda for the Interpretation of Lived Experience.*
Newbury Park, CA: Sage.

Emerson, R. M. (1981). Observational fieldwork. *Annual Review of Sociology* 7:51–
78.

Emerson, R. M. (Ed.)(1983). *Contemporary Field Research: A Collection of Readings*, 1st
ed. Prospect Heights, IL: Waveland.

Emerson, R. M. (Ed.) (2001). *Contemporary Field Research: Perspectives and Formulations* 2nd ed. Prospect Heights, IL: Waveland.

Emerson, R. M., & Pollner M. (1988). On members' responses to researchers' accounts. *Human Organization* 47:89–98.

Emerson, R. M., Fretz, R. I., & Shaw, L. L. (1995). *Writing Ethnographic Fieldnotes.* Chicago: University of Chicago Press.

Emslie, C., Hunt, K., & Watt, G. (2001). Invisible women? Gender, lay beliefs and
heart problems. *Sociology of Health and Illness* 23(2):203–33.

Evans-Pritchard, E. E. (1940). *The Nuer: A Description of the Modes of Livelihood and
Political Institutions of a Nilotic People.* Oxford: Clarendon Press.

Fay, B. (1996). *Contemporary Philosophy of Social Science.* Oxford: Blackwell.

Figlio, K. (1978), Chlorosis and chronic disease in nineteenth-century Britain: The
social constitution of somatic illness in a capitalist society. *Social History* 3: 167-
198

Finch, J. (1986). *Research and Policy: The Uses of Qualitative Methods in Social and Educational Research.* Lewes: Falmer.

Fine, M. (1994). Working the hyphens: reinventing self and other in qualitative research. In N. Denzin & Y. Lincoln (Eds.), *Handbook of Qualitative Research* (pp.
70–82). Thousand Oaks, CA: Sage.

Firestone, W. (1993). Alternative arguments for generalising from data as applied
to qualitative research. *Educational Researcher* 22(4):16–23.

Fisher, S. (1995). *Nursing Wounds: Nurse Practitioners, Doctors, Women Patients and
the Negotiation of Meaning.* New Brunswick, NJ: Rutgers University Press.

Flaherty, M., Denzin, N. K., Manning, P. K., & Snow, D. A. (2002). Review sympo-
sium: Crisis in representation. *Journal of Contemporary Ethnography* 31 (4): 478-
516.

Flick, U. (1992). Triangulation revisited: Strategy of validation or alternative. *Journal for the Theory of Social Behavior* 22(2):175–97.

Foster, F., Lader, D., & Cheesbrough, S. (1997). *Infant Feeding 1995.* London: The
Stationery Office.

Fox, K. V. (1996). Silent voices: A subversive reading of child sexual abuse. In C. Ellis
& A. Bochner (Eds.), *Composing Ethnography: Alternative Forms of Qualitative
Writing* (pp. 330–56). Walnut Creek, CA: Altamira.

Frake, C. (1964). How to ask for a drink in Subanun. *American Anthropologist* 66:27–
32.

Fujimoto, N. (2001). What was that secret? Framing forced disclosures from teen mothers. *Symbolic Interaction* 24(1):1–24.

Gantley, M., Davies, D., & Murcott, A. (1993). Sudden infant death syndrome: Links with infant care practices. *British Medical Journal* 306:6–20.

Garcia, A. and Parmer, P. A. (1999). Misplaced mistrust: The collaborative construction of doubt in 911 emergency calls. *Symbolic Interaction* 22:297–324.

Garfinkel, H. (1967). *Studies in Ethnomethodology*. Englewood Cliffs, NJ: Prentice Hall.

Garfinkel, H. (2002). *Ethnomethodology's Program: Working Out Durkheim's Aphorism*. Lanham, MD: Rowman & Littlefield.

Gitlin, A. D., Siegel, M., & Boru, K. (1989). The politics of method: From leftist ethnography to educative research. *Qualitative Studies in Education* 2(3):237–53.

Glaser, B. G. (1992). *Emergence vs. Forcing: Basics of Grounded Theory Analysis*. Mill Valley, CA: Sociology Press.

Glaser, B. G., & Strauss, A. L. (1965a). The discovery of substantive theory: A basic strategy underlying qualitative research. *American Behavioral Scientist* 8(6):5–12.

Glaser, B. G., & Strauss, A. L. (1965b). *Awareness of Dying*. Chicago: Aldine.

Glaser, B. G., & Strauss, A. L. (1967). *The Discovery of Grounded Theory: Strategies for Qualitative Research*. Chicago: Aldine.

Goffman, E. (1959). *The Presentation of Self in Everyday Life*. Harmondsworth: Penguin.

Goffman, E. (1961). *Asylums*. New York: Doubleday.

Goffman, E. (1969). The insanity of place. *Psychiatry* 32:357–87.

Goffman, E. (1983). Felicity's Condition. *American Journal of Sociology* 9:1–53.

Gold, R. (1969). Roles in sociological field observations. In G. McCall and J. Simmons (Eds.), *Issues in Participant Observation: A Text and Reader* (pp. 30–39). Reading, MA: Addison-Wesley.

Gould, L., Walker, A., Crane, L., & Lidz, C. (1974). *Connections: Notes from the Heroin World*. New Haven, CT: Yale University Press.

Graffam Walker, A. (1986). The verbatim record: The myth and the reality. In S. Fisher & A. Todd (Eds.), *Discourse and Institutional Authority: Medicine, Education and Law* (pp. 205–22). Norwood, NJ: Ablex.

Grbich, C. (1999). *Qualitative Research in Health*. London: Sage.

Greatbatch, D., Heath, C. C., Campion, P., & Luff, P. (1995a). How do desk-top computers affect the doctor-patient interaction? *Family Practice* 12(1):32–36.

Greatbatch, D., Heath, C. C., Luff, P., & Campion, P. (1995b). Conversation analysis: Human-computer interaction and the general practice consultation. In A. Monk & N. Gilbert (Eds.), *Perspectives on Human-Computer Interaction* (pp. 199–222). London: Academic Press.

Greatbatch, D., Luff, P., Heath, C. C., and Campion, P. (1993). Interpersonal communication and human-computer interaction: An examination of computers in medical consultations. *Interacting with Computers* 5:93–216.

Greene, J. (1996). Qualitative evaluation and scientific citizenship. *Evaluation* 2(3):277–89.

Guba, E. G. (1981). Criteria for assessing the trustworthiness of naturalistic inquiries. *Educational Communication and Technology Journal* 29(2):75–91.

Guba, E. G., & Lincoln, Y. S. (1989). *Fourth Generation Evaluation*. Newbury Park, CA: Sage.

Gubrium, J. (1975). *Living and Dying at Murray Manor*. New York: St Martin's.

Gubrium, J., & Buckholdt, D. (1982). *Describing Care: Image and Practice in Rehabilitation*. Cambridge MA: Oelgeschlager, Gunn and Hain.

Guillemin, J. H., & Holmstrom, L. L. (1986). *Mixed Blessings: Intensive Care for Newborns*. New York: Oxford University Press.

Habermann-Little, B. (1991). Qualitative research methodologies: An overview. *Journal of Neuroscience Nursing* 23(3):188–90.

Halloran, J., & Grimes, D. (1995). Application of the focus group methodology to educational program development. *Qualitative Health Research* 5(4):444–53.

Hammersley, M. (1990). *Reading Ethnographic Research*. New York: Longman.

Hammersley, M. (1992a). Ethnography and realism. In M. Hammersley (Ed.) *What's Wrong with Ethnography* (pp. 43–56). London: Routledge.

Hammersley, M. (1992b). Deconstructing the qualitative-quantitative divide. In M. Hammersley (Ed.), *What's Wrong with Ethnography?* (pp. 159–82). London: Routledge.

Hammersley, M. (1992c), On feminist methodology, *Sociology* 26:87–206.

Hammersley, M. (1992d). Some questions about theory in ethnography and history. In M. Hammersley (Ed.), *What's Wrong with Ethnography?* (pp. 32–42). London: Routledge.

Hammersley, M. (1992e). What's wrong with ethnography? The myth of theoretical description. In M. Hammersley (Ed.), *What's Wrong with Ethnography?* (pp. 11–31). London: Routledge.

Hammersley, M. (1992f). The generalisability of ethnography. In M. Hammersley (Ed.), *What's Wrong with Ethnography?* (pp. 85–95). London: Routledge.

Hammersley, M. (1993). *What Is Social Research?* Milton Keynes: Open University Press.

Hammersley, M. (1995). *The Politics of Social Research*. London: Sage.

Hammersley, M., & Atkinson, P. (1995). *Ethnography: Principles in Practice*. London: Routledge.

Harding, S. (1987). *Feminism and Methodology*. Bloomington: Indiana University Press.

Hayek, F. (1945). The use of knowledge in society. *American Economic Review* 55: 519–30.

Hazelgrove, J. (2002). The old faith and the new science: The Nuremberg Code and human experimentation ethics in Britain 1946–73. *Social History of Medicine* 15:109–35.

Heath, C. C. (1992). The delivery and reception of diagnosis in the general practice consultation. In P. Drew & J. Heritage (Eds.), *Talk at Work: Interaction in Institutional Settings* (pp. 235–67). Cambridge: Cambridge University Press.

Heclo, H., & Wildavsky, A. (1974). *The Private Government of Public Money: Community and Policy inside British Politics*. London: Macmillan.

Henwood, K. L., & Pidgeon, N. F. (1992). Qualitative research and psychological theorising. *British Journal of Psychology* 83(1):97–111.

Heritage, J., & Sefi, S. (1992). Dilemmas of advice: Aspects of the delivery and reception of advice in interactions between health visitors and first time mothers. In P. Drew & J. Heritage (Eds.), *Talk at Work: Interaction in Institutional Settings* (pp. 359–417). Cambridge: Cambridge University Press.

Hinds, P. S., Scandrett-Hibden, S., & McAulay, L. S. (1990). Further assessment of a method to estimate reliability and validity of qualitative research findings. *Journal of Advanced Nursing* 15(4):430–35.

Homan, R. (1980). The ethics of covert methods. *British Journal of Sociology* 31(1): 46–59.

House, E. (1990). An ethics of qualitative field studies. In E. Guba (Ed.), *The Paradigm Dialog* (pp. 158–201). Newbury Park, CA: Sage.

Hughes, R. (1998). Considering the vignette technique and its application to a study of drug injecting and HIV risk and safer behaviour. *Sociology of Health and Illness* 20(3):381–400.

Humphreys, L. (1970). *Tearoom Trade*. Chicago: Aldine.

Hunt, K., Emslie, C., & Watt, G. (2000). Barriers rooted in biography: How interpretations of family patterns of heart disease and early life experiences may undermine behavioural change in mid-life. In H. Graham (Ed.), *Understanding Health Inequalities*. Buckingham: Open University Press.

Ianni, F., & Ianni, E. (1972). *A Family Business: Kinship and Social Control in Organised Crime*. London: Routledge.

Imle, M. A., & Atwood, J. R. (1988). Retaining qualitative validity while gaining quantitative reliability and validity: Development of the Transition to Parenthood Concerns Scale. *Ans-Advances in Nursing Science* 11(1):61–75.

Jackson, J. E. (1990). "I am a fieldnote": Fieldnotes as a symbol of professional identity. In R. Sanjek (Ed.), *Fieldnotes: The Makings of Anthropology* (pp. 3–33). Ithaca, NY: Cornell University Press.

Janesick, V. (1994). The dance of qualitative research design: metaphor, methodolatory and meaning. In N. Denzin & Y. Lincoln (Eds.), *A Handbook of Qualitative Research,* 1st ed. (pp. 209–19). Thousand Oaks, CA: Sage.

Jefferson, G. (1984). Transcript notation. In J. M. Atkinson & J. C. Heritage (Eds.) *Structures of Social Action: Studies in Conversation Analysis* (pp. ix–xvi). Cambridge: Cambridge University Press.

Jeffery, R. (1979). Normal rubbish: Deviant patients in casualty departments, *Sociology of Health and Illness* 1(1):90–107.

Jensen, G. M. (1989). Qualitative methods in physical therapy research: A form of disciplined inquiry. *Physical Therapy* 69(6):492–500.

Jick, T. D. (1979). Mixing qualitative and quantitative methods: Triangulation in action. *Administrative Science Quarterly* 24:602–11.

Jones, J. H. (1981). *Bad Blood: The Tuskegee Syphilis Experiment*. New York: Free Press.

Josselson, R. (1996). On writing other people's lives: Self-analytic reflections of a narrative researcher. In R. Josselson (Ed.), *Ethics and Process in the Narrative Study of Lives* (pp. 60–71). Thousand Oaks, CA: Sage.

Junker, B. (1960). *Field Work: An Introduction to the Social Sciences*. Chicago: University of Chicago Press.

Kaplan, B. (1986). Impact of a clinical laboratory computer system: Users' perceptions. In B. Blum & M. Jorgensen (Eds.), *Medinfo 86: Fifth World Congress on
   Medical Informatics* (pp. 1057–61). Amsterdam: North Holland.

Kaplan, B. (1987). Initial impact of a clinical laboratory computer system: Themes
   common to expectations and actualities. *Journal of Medical Systems* 11:37–47.

Kaplan, B., & Duchon, D. (1988). Combining qualitative and quantitative methods
   in information systems research: A case study. *MIS Quarterly* 12:571–86.

Kaplan, B., & Duchon, D. (1989). A job orientation model of impact on work seven
   months post implementation. In B. Barber, D. Cao, D. Qin, & G. Wagner (Eds.),
   Medinfo 89: Sixth World Congress on Medical Informatics (pp. 1051–55). Amsterdam: North Holland.

Kelle, U., & Laurie, H. (1995). Computer use in qualitative research and issues of
   validity. In U. Kelle (Ed.), *Computer-Aided Qualitative Data Analysis* (pp. 19–28).
   London: Sage.

Kelly, M., & May, D. (1982). Good and bad patients: A review of the literature and
   a theoretical critique. *Journal of Advanced Nursing* 7:147–56.

King, L. (1954). What is disease? *Philosophy of Science* 21:193–203.

Kleinman, S. (1993). The textual turn. *Contemporary Sociology* 22(1):11–13.

Kleinman, S., Stenross, B., & McMahon, M. (1994). Privileging fieldwork over
   interviews: Consequences for identity and practice. *Symbolic Interaction*
   17(1):37–50.

Klockars, C. B. (1974) *The Professional Fence*. New York: Free Press.

Klockars, C. B. (1979). Dirty hands and deviant subjects. In C. Klockars & F.
   O'Connor (Eds.), *Deviance and Decency: The Ethics of Research with Human Subjects* (pp. 261-82). Beverly Hills, CA: Sage.

Kolker, A. (1996). Thrown overboard: The human costs of health care rationing. In
   C. Ellis & A. Bochner (Eds.), *Composing Ethnography: Alternative Forms of Qualitative Writing* (pp. 132–59). Walnut Creek, CA: Altamira.

Lather, P. (1986). Issues of validity in openly ideological research. *Interchange*,
   17(4):63–84.

Lather, P. (1991). *Getting Smart: Feminist Research and Pedagogy with/in the Postmodern*.
   New York: Routledge.

Lather, P. (1993). Fertile obsession: Validity after post-structuralism. *Sociological
   Quarterly*, 34(4):673–93.

Latour, B. and Woolgar, S. (1979) *Laboratory Life: The Social Construction of Scientific
   Facts*. Beverly Hills: Sage

Lauritzen, S. O., (1997). Notions of child health: Mothers' accounts of health in their
   young babies. *Sociology of Health and Illness* 19(4):436–56.

LeCompte, M., & Goetz, J. P. (1982). Problems of reliability and validity in ethnographic research. *Review of Educational Research* 52:31–60.

Lewis, O. (1961). *The Children of Sánchez: Autobiography of a Mexican Family*. New York:
   Modern Library.

Lieblich, A. (1996). Some unforeseen outcomes of narrative research. In R. Josselson
   (Ed.), *Ethics and Process in the Narrative Study of Lives* (pp. 172–184). Thousand
   Oaks, CA: Sage.

Lifton, R. J. (1986). *The Nazi Doctors: Medical Killing and the Psychology of Genocide*.
   New York: Basic Books.

Light, D. (1980). *Becoming Psychiatrists: An Inside Account of the Psychiatric Residency with Implications for Both the Profession and the Patient.* New York: W. W. Norton.

Lincoln, Y. (1990). The making of a constructivist: A remembrance of transformations past. In E. Guba (Ed.), *The Paradigm Dialog* (pp. 67–87). Newbury Park, CA: Sage.

Lincoln, Y. S., & Guba, E. G. (1985). *Naturalistic Inquiry.* Newbury Park, CA: Sage.

Lincoln, Y. S., & Guba, E. G. (2000). Paradigmatic controversies, contradictions, and emerging confluences. In N. Denzin & Y. Lincoln (Eds.), *Handbook of Qualitative Research,* 2nd ed. (pp. 163–88). Thousand Oaks, CA: Sage.

Lindlof, T. R. (1995). *Qualitative Communication Research Methods.* London: Sage.

Lofland, J. (1967). Notes on naturalism. *Kansas Journal of Sociology* 3(2):45–61.

Lofland, J. (1971). *Analyzing Social Settings: A Guide to Qualitative Observation and Analysis.* Belmont, CA: Wadsworth.

Lofland, J. (1976). *Doing Social Life: The Qualitative Study of Human Interaction in Natural Settings.* New York: Wiley.

Lonkila, M. (1995). Grounded theory as an emerging paradigm for qualitative data analysis. In U. Kelle (Ed.), *Computer-Aided Qualitative Data Analysis* (pp. 41–51). London: Sage.

Lyttinen, K. (1987). Different perspectives on information systems: Problems and solutions. *ACM Computing Surveys* 19:5–46.

Lyttinen, K., & Hirschheim, R. (1987). Information systems failure: A survey and classification of empirical literature. *Oxford Surveys in Information Technology* 4:257–309.

MacIntyre, A. (1982). Risk, harm and benefits assessments as instruments of moral evaluation. In T. Beauchamp, R. Faden, R. Wallace, & L. Walters (Eds.), *Ethical Issues in Social Science Research* (pp. 193–214). Baltimore, MD: Johns Hopkins University Press.

Macintyre, S. (1978). Some notes on record taking and making in an antenatal clinic. *Sociological Review* 26:595–611.

Malinowski, B. (1922). *Argonauts of the Western Pacific.* London: George Routledge & Sons.

Malinowski, B. (1967). *A Diary in the Strict Sense of the Term.* London: Routledge & Kegan Paul.

Mangione-Smith, R., Stivers, T., Elliott, M., McDonald, L., & Heritage, J. (2003). On-line commentary during the physical examination: A communication tool for avoiding inappropriate antibiotic prescribing? *Social Science & Medicine* 56(2):313-20.

Manzo, J. F., Blonder, L. X., & Burns, A. F. (1995). The social-interactional organisation of narrative and narrating among stroke patients and their spouses. *Sociology of Health and Illness* 17(3):307–27.

Markens, S., Browner, C. H., & Press, N. (1999). "Because of the risks": How U.S. pregnant women account for refusing perinatal screening. *Social Science and Medicine* 492:359–69.

Marshall, C. (1985). Appropriate criteria of the trustworthiness and goodness for qualitative research on educational organisations. *Quality and Quantity* 19: 353–73.

Mathieson, C. M., & Stam, H. J. (1995). Renegotiating identity: Cancer narratives. *Sociology of Health and Illness* 17(3):283–306.

Maynard, D. (1989). On the ethnography and analysis of discourse in institutional settings. *Perspectives on Social Problems* 1:127–46.

Maynard, D. (1991a). The perspective-display series and the delivery and receipt of diagnostic news. In D. Boden & D. Zimmerman (Eds.), *Talk and Social Structure: Studies in Ethnomethodology and Conversation Analysis* (pp. 164–92). Cambridge: Polity.

Maynard, D. (1991b). Interaction and asymmetry in clinical discourse. *American Journal of Sociology* 97:448–95.

Maynard, D. (1992). On clinicians co-implicating recipients' perspective in the deliv-ery of diagnostic news. In P. Drew & J. Heritage (Eds.), *Talk at Work: Interaction in Institutional Settings* (pp. 331–58). Cambridge: Cambridge University Press.

McCorkel, J. A. (1998). Going to the crackhouse: Critical space as a form of resistance in total institutions and everyday life. *Symbolic Interaction* 23(1):227–52.

McCracken, G. (1988). *The Long Interview.* Newbury Park, CA: Sage.

McHugh, P. S. (1968). *Defining the Situation; The Organization of Meaning in Social Interaction.* Indianapolis: Bobbs-Merrill.

McKeganey, N., & Bloor, M. (1991). Spotting the invisible man: The influence of male gender on fieldwork relations. *British Journal of Sociology* 42:195–210.

Mead, G. H. (1934). *Mind, Self and Society from the Standpoint of a Social Behaviorist.* Chicago: University of Chicago Press.

Melia, K. (1997). Producing "plausible stories": Interviewing student nurses. In G. Miller & R. Dingwall (Eds.), *Context and Method in Qualitative Research* (pp. 26–36). London: Sage.

Merriam, S. (1988). *Case Study Research in Education: A Qualitative Approach.* San Francisco, CA: Jossey Bass.

Messenger, J. (1989). *Inis Beag Revisited: The Anthropologist as Participant Observer.* Salem, WI: Sheffield.

Meyer, J. W., & Rowan, B. (1977). Institutionalized organizations: Formal structure as myth and ceremony. *American Journal of Sociology* 83 (2): 340-63.

Mienczakowski, J., & Morgan, S. (1993). *Busting: The Challenge of the Drought Spirit.* Brisbane: Griffith University Reprographics.

Mies, M. (1983). Towards a methodology for feminist research. In G. Bowles & R. Duelli Klein (Eds.), *Theories of Women's Studies.* London: Routledge & Kegan Paul.

Mill, J. S. (1973). *A System of Logic Ratiocinative and Inductive: Being a Connected View of the Principles of Evidence and the Methods of Scientific Investigation.* Books I–III and Appendices. Toronto: University of Toronto Press; London: Routledge & Kegan Paul.

Miller, G. (1997). *Becoming Miracle Workers: Language and Meaning in Brief Therapy.* Hawthorne, NY: Aldine de Gruyter.

Miller, G., & Silverman D. (1995). Troubles talk and counseling discourse: A comparative study. *Sociological Quarterly* 36(4):725–47.

Millman, M. (1976). *The Unkindest Cut: Life in the Backrooms of Medicine.* New York: William Morrow.

Mills, C. Wright (1940). Situated action and the vocabulary of motives. *American Sociological Review* 6:904–13.

Mishler, E. G. (1979). Meaning in context: Is there any other kind? *Harvard Educational Review* 49:1–19.

Mitchell, R. G. (1993). *Secrecy and Fieldwork*. Newbury Park, CA: Sage.

Mizrahi, T. (1986). *Getting Rid of Patients: Contradictions in the Socialization of Physicians*. New Brunswick, NJ: Rutgers University Press.

Morgan, D. (1992). Doctor-care giver relationships: An exploration using focus groups. In B. Crabtree & W. Miller (Eds.), *Doing Qualitative Research*. Thousand Oaks, CA: Sage.

Morgan, D. H. J. (1972). The British Association scandal: The effect of publicity on a sociological investigation. *Sociological Review* 20(2):185–206.

Morgan, M., & Watkins C. J. (1988). Managing hypertension: Beliefs and responses to medication among cultural groups. *Sociology of Health and Illness* 10(4):561–78.

Morse, J. (1994). Designing funded qualitative research. In N. Denzin & Y. Lincoln (Eds.), *A Handbook Of Qualitative Research*, 1st ed. (pp. 220-35). Thousand Oaks, CA: Sage.

Munhall, P. L. (1993). Epistemology in nursing. In P. L. Munhall & C. Oiler Boyd (Eds.), *Nursing Research: A Qualitative Perspective*, 2nd ed. (pp. 39–65). New York: National League for Nursing.

Murphy, E. A. (1999). Breast is best: Infant feeding and maternal deviance. *Sociology of Health and Illness* 21(2):187–208.

Murphy, E. A. (2000). Risk, responsibility and rhetoric in infant feeding. *Journal of Contemporary Ethnography* 29(3):291–325.

Murphy, E., & Dingwall, R. (2001). The ethics of ethnography. In P. Atkinson, A. Coffey, S. Delamont, J. Lofland, & L. Lofland (Eds.), *Handbook of Ethnography* (pp. 339–51). London: Sage.

Murphy, E., Dingwall, R., Greatbatch, D., Parker, S., & Watson, P. (1998) Qualitative research methods in health technology assessment: A review of the literature. *Health Technology Assessment* 2, No.16, Southampton: National Coordinating Centre for Health Technology Assessment.

Murray, S. B. (2000). Getting paid in smiles: The gendering of child care work. *Symbolic Interaction* 23(2):135–60.

Nolan, M., & Behi, R. (1995). Triangulation: The best of all worlds? *British Journal of Nursing* 4(14):829–32.

Norris, P. (2001). How "we" are different from "them": Occupational boundary maintenance in the treatment of musculo-skeletal problems. *Sociology of Health and Illness* 23(1):24–43.

North, D., Davis, P., & Powell, A. (1995). Patient responses to benzodiazepine medication: A typology of adaptive repertoires developed by long-term users. *Sociology of Health and Illness* 17(5):632–50.

Oakley, A. (1980). *Women Confined: Towards A Sociology of Childbirth*. Oxford: Martin Robertson.

Oakley, A. (1998). Gender, methodology and people's ways of knowing: Some problems with feminism and the paradigm debate in social science. *Sociology* 32(4):707–31.

Oiler Boyd, C. (1993a). Combining qualitative and quantitative approaches. In P. L. Munhall & C. Oiler Boyd (Eds.), *Nursing Research: A Qualitative Perspective* (pp. 454-75). New York: National League for Nursing.

Oiler Boyd, C. (1993b). Philosophical foundations of qualitative research. In P. L. Munhall & C. Oiler Boyd (Eds.), *Nursing Research: A Qualitative Perspective* (pp. 66-93). New York: National League for Nursing.

Paget, M. A. (1983). Experience and knowledge. *Human Studies* 6:67–90.

Paget, M. A. (1990). Performing the text. *Journal Of Contemporary Ethnography* 19:136–55.

Palmer, V. (1928). *Field Studies in Sociology*. Chicago: University of Chicago Press.

Parsons, T. (1951). *The Social System*. London: Routledge & Kegan Paul.

Patai, D. (1991). U.S. academics and third world women: Is ethical research possible? In S. Gluck & D. Patai (Eds.), *Women's Words and the Feminist Practice of Oral History* (pp. 137–53). New York: Routledge.

Patton, M. Q. (1980). *Qualitative Evaluation Methods*. Newbury Park CA: Sage.

Patton, M. Q. (1990). *Qualitative Evaluation And Research Methods,* 2nd ed. Newbury Park, CA: Sage.

Penslar, R. L., & Porter, J. P. (Eds.) (1993). *Protecting Human Research Subjects: Institutional Review Board Guidebook* (2nd ed.). Washington, DC: Office for Human Research Protections. Available at http://ohrp.osophs.dhhs.gov/irb/irb_guidebook.htm.

Phillips, D.C. (1987). Validity in qualitative research: Why the worry about warrant will not wane. *Education and Urban Society* 20:9–24.

Pill, R. (1995). Fitting the method to the question: The quantitative or qualitative approach? In R. Jones & A. L. Kinmonth (Eds.), *Critical Reading for Primary Care* (pp. 42–58). Oxford: Oxford University Press.

Pilnick, A. (1999). "Patient counseling" by pharmacists: Advice, information or instruction? *Sociological Quarterly* 40:613–22.

Pilnick, A., & Hindmarsh, J. (1999). "When you wake up, it'll all be over": Communication in the anaesthetic room. *Symbolic Interaction* 22:345–60.

Platt, J. (1996). *History of Sociological Research Methods in America 1920–1960*. Cambridge: Cambridge University Press.

Pollner, M. (1975). "The very coinage of your brain": The anatomy of reality disjunctures. *Philosophy of the Social Sciences* 5:411–30.

Polsky, N. (1971). *Hustlers, Beats and Others*. Harmondsworth: Penguin.

Pope, C. (2002). Contingency in everyday surgical work. *Sociology of Health and Illness* 24:369–84.

Popper, K. (1959). *The Logic of Scientific Discovery.* London: Hutchinson.

Power, M. (1997). *The Audit Society: Rituals of Verification*. Oxford: Oxford University Press.

Price, J. (1996). Snakes in the swamp: Ethical issues in qualitative research. In R. Josselson (Ed.), *Ethics and Process in the Narrative Study of Lives* (pp. 207-15). Thousand Oaks, CA: Sage.

Prior, L. (1985). Making sense of mortality. *Sociology of Health and Illness* 7: 167–90.

Prior, L. (1988). The architecture of the hospital: A study of spatial-organization and medical knowledge. *British Journal of Sociology* 39:86–113.

Punch, M. (1994). Politics and ethics in qualitative research. In N. Denzin & Y. Lincoln (Eds.), *Handbook of Qualitative Research,* 1st ed. (pp. 83–97). Thousand Oaks, CA: Sage.

Rawlings, B. (1989). Coming clean: The symbolic use of clinical hygiene in a hospital sterilising unit. *Sociology of Health and Illness* 11:279–93.

Rhodes, T., & Cusick, L. (2000). Love and intimacy in relationship risk management. *Sociology of Health and Illness* 22(1):1–26.

Richardson, L. (1988). The collective story: Postmodernism and the writing of sociology. *Sociological Focus* 21(3):199–207.

Richardson, L. (1992). The consequences of poetic representation. In C. Ellis & M. Flaherty (Eds.), *Investigating Subjectivity: Research on Lived Experience* (pp. 125–37). Newbury Park, CA: Sage.

Richardson, S., Dohrenwend, B., & Klein, D. (1966). *Interviewing: Its Forms and Functions.* New York: Basic Books.

Roman, L., & Apple M. (1990). Is naturalism a move away from positivism? Materialist and feminist approaches to subjectivity in ethnographic research. In E. Eisner & A. Peshkin (Eds.), *Qualitative Inquiry in Education: The Continuing Debate* (pp. 38–73). New York: Teachers' College Press.

Ronai, C. R. (1992). The reflexive self through narrative. In C. Ellis & M. Flaherty (Eds.), *Investigating Subjectivity: Research on Lived Experience* (pp. 103–24). Newbury Park, CA: Sage.

Ronai, C. R. (1996). My mother is mentally retarded. In C. Ellis & A. Bochner (Eds.), *Composing Ethnography: Alternative Forms of Qualitative Writing* (pp. 109–31). Walnut Creek, CA: Altamira.

Rosenau, P. M. (1992). *Postmodernism and the Social Sciences: Insights, Inroads and Intrusions.* Princeton, NJ: Princeton University Press.

Roth, J. A. (1957). Ritual and magic in the control of contagion. *American Sociological Review* 22:310–14.

Roth, J. A., & Douglas, D. (1983). *No Appointment Necessary: The Hospital Emergency Department in the Medical Services World.* New York: Irvington.

Rothman, D. J. (1993). *Strangers at the Bedside. A History of How Law and Bioethics Transformed Medical Decision Making.* New York: Basic Books.

Sacks, H. (1995). *Lectures on Conversation* (2 vols.). Oxford: Blackwell.

Sandelowski, M. (1986). The problem of rigor in qualitative research. *Ans-Advances in Nursing Science* 8(3):27–37.

Sanders, C. R. (1995). Stranger than fiction: Insights and pitfalls in post-modern ethnography. In N. Denzin (Ed.), *Studies in Symbolic Interaction, 17* (pp. 89–104). Greenwich, CT: JAI.

Sanjek, R. (Ed.) (1990). *Fieldnotes: The Makings of Anthropology.* Ithaca, NY: Cornell University Press.

Schatzman, L., & Strauss, A. (1973). *Field Research: Strategies for a Natural Sociology.* Englewood Cliffs, NJ: Prentice Hall.

Schegloff, E. (1991). Reflections on talk and social structure. In D. Boden & D. Zimmerman (Eds.), *Talk and Social Structure* (pp. 44–70). Cambridge: Polity.

Schegloff, E. (1997). Whose text? Whose context? *Discourse and Society* 8:165–88.

Scheper-Hughes, N. (1982). *Saints, Scholars and Schizophrenics: Mental Illness in Rural Ireland.* Berkeley: University of California Press.

Schofield, J. (1993). Increasing the generalizability of qualitative research. In M.

Hammersley (Ed.), *Social Research: Philosophy, Politics and Practice* (pp. 200-25). London: Sage.

Schutz, A. (1962). *Collected Papers*, vol. 1: *The Problem Of Social Reality*. Edited By M. Natanson. The Hague: Martinus Nijhoff.

Schwandt, T. (1997). *Qualitative Inquiry: A Dictionary of Terms*. Thousand Oaks, CA: Sage.

Scott, M., & Lyman, S. (1968). Accounts. *American Sociological Review* 33:46–62.

Seale, C. (1995). Dying alone. *Sociology of Health and Illness* 17(3):376–92.

Seale, C. (1999). *The Quality of Qualitative Research*. London: Sage.

Secker, J., Wimbush, E., Watson, J., & Milburn, K. (1995). Qualitative methods in health promotion research: Some criteria for quality. *Health Education Journal* 54:74–87.

Seidel, J. (1991). Method and madness in the application of computer technology to qualitative data analysis. In N. G. Fielding & R. M. Lee (Eds.), *Using Computers in Qualitative Research* (pp. 107–16). London: Sage.

Shaffir, W., Stebbins, R., & Turowetz, A. (1980). *Fieldwork Experience: Qualitative Approaches to Social Research*. New York: St Martin's.

Sharrock, W. (1979). Portraying the professional relationship. In D. Anderson (Ed.) *Health Education in Practice* (pp. 125–46). London: Croom Helm.

Shaw, C.R. (1966). *The Jack-Roller : A Delinquent Boy's Own Story*. Chicago: University of Chicago Press.

Sheehan, E. (1993). The student of culture and the ethnography of Irish intellectuals. In C. Brettell (Ed.), *When They Read What We Write: The Politics of Ethnography* (pp.75-89). Westport, CT: Bergen and Garvey.

Silverman, D. (1985). *Qualitative Methodology and Sociology*. Aldershot: Gower.

Silverman, D. (1989). Telling convincing stories: A plea for cautious positivism in case studies. In B. Glassner & J. D. Moreno (Eds.), *The Qualitative-Quantitative Distinction in the Social Sciences* (pp.57-77). Dordrecht: Kluwer Academic.

Silverman, D. (1993). *Interpreting Qualitative Data: Methods for Analysing Talk, Text and Interaction*. London: Sage.

Silverman, D. (1997). *Discourses of Counselling: HIV Counselling as Social Interaction*. London: Sage.

Silverman, D. (2000). *Doing Qualitative Research: A Practical Handbook*. London: Sage.

Silverman, D., Bor, R., Miller, R., & Goldman, E. (1992). Obviously the advice is then to keep to safer sex: Advice giving and advice reception in AIDS Counselling. In P. Aggleton, P. Davies, & G. Hart (Eds.), *AIDS: Rights, Risks and Reason* (pp. 174-91). London: Falmer.

Skrtic, T., Guba, E. G., & Knowlton, H. (1985). *Special Education in Rural America: Interorganizational Special Education Programming in Rural Areas*. Washington, DC: Department Of Education, National Institute Of Education.

Smith, H. (1975). *Strategies of Social Research: The Methodological Imagination*. London: Prentice Hall.

Smith, J. K. (1984). The problem of criteria for judging interpretive inquiry. *Educational Evaluation and Policy Analysis* 6:379–91.

Smith, J. K. (1985). Social reality as mind-dependent versus mind-independent and the interpretation of test validity. *Journal of Research and Development in Education* 19(1):1–9.

Solzhenitsyn, A. (1971). *Cancer Ward*. Harmondsworth: Penguin.

Stake, R. E. (1995). *The Art of Case Study Research*. Thousand Oaks, CA: Sage.

Stein, L. I. (1967). The doctor-nurse game. *Archives of General Psychiatry* 16:699–703.

Stein, L. I., Watts, D. T., & Howell, T. (1990). The doctor-nurse game revisited. *New England Journal of Medicine* 322: 546-549.

Stimson, G., &. Webb, B. (1975). *Going to See the Doctor*. London: Routledge & Kegan Paul.

Strauss, A., &. Corbin, J. (1990). *Basics of Qualitative Research: Grounded Theory Products and Techniques*. Newbury Park, CA: Sage.

Strauss, A., Schatzman, L., Bucher, R., Erlich, D., & Sabshin, M. (1964). *Psychiatric Ideologies and Institutions*. Glencoe, IL: Free Press.

Strong, P.M. (1983) The Rivals: An essay on the sociological trades. In R. Dingwall & P.S.C. Lewis, (Eds.), *The Sociology of the Professions: Lawyers, Doctors and Others* (pp. 59–77). London: Macmillan.

Strong, P.M. (1988). Qualitative sociology in the UK. *Qualitative Sociology* 11:13–28.

Sudnow, D. (1967). *Passing On: The Social Organization of Dying*. Englewood Cliffs, NJ: Prentice Hall.

Svensson, R. (1996). The interplay between doctors and nurses: A negotiated order perspective. *Sociology of Health and Illness* 18(3):379–98.

Taylor, S. J. (2000). "You're not just a retard, you're just wise": Disability, social identity and family networks. *Journal of Contemporary Ethnography* 29(1):58–92.

ten Have, P. (1991). Talk and institution: a reconsideration of the "asymmetry" of doctor-patient interaction. In D. Boden & D. Zimmerman (Eds.), *Talk and Social Structure: Studies in Ethnomethodology and Conversation Analysis* (pp. 138–63). Cambridge: Polity.

Tillmann-Healy, L. M. (1996). A secret life in a culture of thinness: reflections on body, food and bulimia. In C. Ellis, & A. Bochner (Eds.), *Composing Ethnography: Alternative Forms of Qualitative Writing* (pp. 76–108). Walnut Creek, CA: Altamira.

Timmermans, S. (1995). *Cui Bono?* Institutional review board ethics and ethnographic research. *Studies in Symbolic Interaction 19* (pp. 153–73). Greenwich, CT: JAI.

Timmermans, S. (1999). *Sudden Death and the Myth of CPR*. Philadelphia: Temple University Press.

Todd, A. (1989). *Intimate Adversaries: Cultural Conflict between Doctors and Women Patients*. Philadelphia: University of Pennsylvania Press.

Trend, M. G. (1979). On the reconciliation of qualitative and quantitative analyses. In C. S. Reichardt & T. D. Cook (Eds.), *Qualitative and Quantitative Methods in Evaluation Research* (pp. 68-86). Beverly Hills, CA: Sage.

Tyler, S. A. (1986). Post-modern ethnography: From document of the occult to occult document. In J. Clifford & C. Marcus (Eds.), *Writing Culture: The Poetics and Politics of Ethnography* (pp. 122-40). Berkeley: University of California Press.

Van Maanen, J. (1988). *Tales of the Field: On Writing Ethnography*. Chicago: University of Chicago Press.

Vidich, A., & Bensman, J. (1958). Freedom and responsibility in research. *Human Organization* 17:1–7.

Vidich, A., & Bensman, J. (1964). The Springdale case: Academic bureaucrats and sensitive townspeople. In A. Vidich, J. Bensman, & M. Stein (Eds.), *Reflections on Community Studies* (pp. 313-49). New York: John Wiley.

Voysey, M. (1975). *A Constant Burden: The Reconstitution of Family Life.* London: Routledge & Kegan Paul.

Waitzkin, H. (1991). *The Politics of Medical Encounters.* New Haven, CT: Yale University Press.

Walker, M. (1989). Analysing qualitative data: Ethnography and the evaluation of medical education. *Medical Education* 23(6):498-503.

Wallace, W. (1978). An overview of elements in the scientific process. In J. Bynner & K. Stribley (Eds.), *Social Research: Principles and Procedures* (pp. 4-10). London: Longman, in association with Open University Press.

Warren, C. A. B. (1988). *Gender Issues in Field Research.* Newbury Park, CA: Sage.

Wax, M., & Cassell J. (1979). Fieldwork, ethics and politics: The wider context. In M. Wax and J. Cassell (Eds.), *Federal Regulations: Ethical Issues and Social Research* (pp. 85-102). Boulder, CO: Westview.

Weber, M. (1947) *The Theory of Social and Economic Organization* (Trans. A. M. Henderson and Talcott Parsons, (Ed.), with an introduction by Talcott Parsons). Glencoe, IL: Free Press.

West, C. (1984a). When the doctor is a "lady": Power, status and gender in physician-patient encounters. *Symbolic Interaction* 7:87-106.

West, C. (1984b). *Routine Complications: Troubles in Talk between Doctors and Patients.* Bloomington, IN: Indiana University Press.

White, A., Freeth, S., & O'Brien, M. (1992). *Infant Feeding 1990.* London: HMSO.

Whyte, W. F. (1980). Interviewing in field research. In R. G. Burgess (Ed.), *Field Research: A Sourcebook and Field Manual* (pp. 111-22). London: Allen and Unwin.

Wiener, C. (2000). *The Elusive Quest: Accountability in Hospitals.* Hawthorne, NY: Aldine de Gruyter.

Wiseman, J. (1970). *Stations of the Lost: The Treatment of Skid Row Alcoholics.* Englewood Cliffs, NJ: Prentice-Hall.

Wolpe, P.R. (1998). The triumph of autonomy in American bioethics: A sociological view. In R. DeVries & J. Subedi (Eds.) *Bioethics and Society: Constructing the Ethical Enterprise* (pp. 38-59). Upper Saddle River, NJ: Prentice Hall.

Wong, L. (1998). The ethics of rapport: Institutional safeguards, resistance and betrayal. *Qualitative Inquiry* 4:178-99.

Yoels, W. C., & Clair, J. M. (1995). Laughter in the clinic: Humor as social organization. *Symbolic Interaction* 18(1):39-58.

Zerubavel, E. (1979). *Patterns of Time in Hospital Life.* Chicago: University of Chicago Press.

Index